Professionalism, Professional Values and Ethics in Nursing

Professionalism, Professional Values and Ethics in Nursing

As per the Revised Syllabus for BSc Nursing

Suresh K Sharma PhD MSc (N) FNRS RN (USA)
Professor and Principal
College of Nursing
All India Institute of Medical Sciences (AIIMS)
Jodhpur, Rajasthan, India

Asha P Shetty PhD MSc (N) RN
Professor and Principal
College of Nursing
All India Institute of Medical Sciences (AIIMS)
Bhubaneswar, Odisha, India

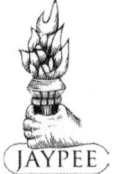

JAYPEE BROTHERS MEDICAL PUBLISHERS
The Health Sciences Publisher
New Delhi | London

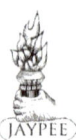

Jaypee Brothers Medical Publishers (P) Ltd

Headquarters
Jaypee Brothers Medical Publishers (P) Ltd
EMCA House, 23/23-B
Ansari Road, Daryaganj
New Delhi 110 002, India
Landline: +91-11-23272143
+91-11-23272703, +91-11-23282021
+91-11-23245672
Email: jaypee@jaypeebrothers.com

Corporate Office
Jaypee Brothers Medical Publishers (P) Ltd
4838/24, Ansari Road, Daryaganj
New Delhi 110 002, India
Phone: +91-11-43574357
Fax: +91-11-43574314
Email: jaypee@jaypeebrothers.com

Overseas Office
J.P. Medical Ltd
83 Victoria Street, London
SW1H 0HW (UK)
Phone: +44 20 3170 8910
Email: info@jpmedpub.com

EU GPSR Authorised Representative
Logos Europe, 9 rue Nicolas Poussin
17000, La Rochelle, France
Phone: +33 (0) 6 67 93 73 78
E-mail: Contact@logoseurope.eu

Website: www.jaypeebrothers.com
Website: www.jaypeedigital.com

© 2023, Jaypee Brothers Medical Publishers

The views and opinions expressed in this book are solely those of the original contributor(s)/author(s) and do not necessarily represent those of editor(s) and publisher of the book.

All rights reserved. No part of this publication may be reproduced, stored or transmitted in any form or by any means, electronic, mechanical, photocopying, recording or otherwise, without the prior permission in writing of the publishers.

All brand names and product names used in this book are trade names, service marks, trademarks or registered trademarks of their respective owners. The publisher is not associated with any product or vendor mentioned in this book.

Medical knowledge and practice change constantly. This book is designed to provide accurate, authoritative information about the subject matter in question. However, readers are advised to check the most current information available on procedures included and check information from the manufacturer of each product to be administered, to verify the recommended dose, formula, method and duration of administration, adverse effects and contraindications. It is the responsibility of the practitioner to take all appropriate safety precautions. Neither the publisher nor the author(s)/editor(s) assume any liability for any injury and/or damage to persons or property arising from or related to use of material in this book.

This book is sold on the understanding that the publisher is not engaged in providing professional medical services. If such advice or services are required, the services of a competent medical professional should be sought.

Every effort has been made where necessary to contact holders of copyright to obtain permission to reproduce copyright material. If any have been inadvertently overlooked, the publisher will be pleased to make the necessary arrangements at the first opportunity.

Inquiries for bulk sales may be solicited at: jaypee@jaypeebrothers.com

Professionalism, Professional Values and Ethics in Nursing

First Edition: **2023**

ISBN: 978-93-5465-965-2

Contributors

Ms Biji P Varkey BScN
Nursing Officer, Directorate of Health Services
Government of Kerala, India

Mr Deepak MScN
Associate Professor, College of Nursing
SGT University, Gurugram, Haryana, India

Mr Jaison Joseph MScN
Lecturer (Jr), College of Nursing
Pandit Bhagwat Dayal Sharma University of Health Sciences
Rohtak, Haryana, India

Dr Rakhi Gaur PhD
Assistant Professor
College of Nursing
All India Institute of Medical Sciences
Deoghar, Jharkhand, India

Mrs R Beutlin MScN
Assistant Professor
The Salvation Army Catherine Booth College of Nursing
Nagercoil, Chennai, India

Dr Shiv Kumar Mudgal PhD
Assistant Professor
College of Nursing
All India Institute of Medical Sciences
Deoghar, Jharkhand, India

Ms Suvashri Sasmal
Nursing Officer
Employees' State Insurance (ESI) Hospital
Kolkata, West Bengal, India

Dr T Johnsy Rani PhD
Senior Lecturer, Villa College, QI Campus
Rahdhebai Hingun, Male, Maldives

Ms Urvashi Goyal BScN
Nursing Officer
All India Institute of Medical Sciences
Bilaspur, Himachal Pradesh, India

Preface

Nursing has merged as a profession which is a science and an art. It is said to be a very noble profession because it requires dedication and commitment to caring for patients with passion and compassion. Apart from these, nursing is indeed a very profitable career and has international scope as well. Nursing has changed from an occupation into a profession through the recent increase in professional independence with the development of definitions for roles and performances.

Professionalism has become one of the important basics in nursing due to the gradual development of educational standards and professional certificates. Nurses are the largest group of healthcare workers, and their professional abilities play a critical part in the development of a functional healthcare system.

This textbook *Professionalism, Professional Values and Ethics in Nursing* is a modest attempt to bring about the basic principles of professionalism in a simple and user-friendly manner by incorporating the attributes or the expected fundamental qualities of nursing professionals. It has been ensured that each basic principle is simply defined and discussed with its application to nursing practices. Each topic of the content is presented in a simple and lucid manner by using illustrations and examples from healthcare and nursing practice areas. The content of this textbook will fully meet the needs of the nursing students studying in the Basic BSc Nursing program since it is designed according to the revised syllabus of the Indian Nursing Council, New Delhi. In addition, it will also be useful for nurses planning for different competitive examinations for jobs or higher studies.

Suresh K Sharma
Asha P Shetty

Contents

Unit 1: Professionals in Nursing

Chapter 1: Profession and Professionalism 3
T Johnsy Rani, R Beutlin
- Profession *3*
- Criteria of a Profession *6*
- Nursing as a Profession *8*
- Characteristics of the Nursing Profession *13*
- Professionalism *16*
- Challenges of Professionalism *24*

Chapter 2: Professional Conduct 36
Biji P Varkey, Deepak
- Professional Conduct *36*
- Ethical Principles and Professional Conduct *40*
- Adherence to Policies, Rules, and Regulations of the Institutions *43*
- Professional Etiquettes and Behaviors *44*
- Professional Grooming: Uniform, Dress Code *45*
- Professional Boundaries: Professional Relationship with the Patients, Caregivers, and Team Members *47*

Chapter 3: Regulatory Bodies and Professional Organization 51
Urvashi Goyal, Jaison Joseph
- Regulatory Bodies: Roles and Responsibilities *51*
- Professional Organization *53*
- International Professional Organizations *54*
- Indian Professional Nursing Organizations *56*

Unit 2: Professional Values

Chapter 4: Professional Values 63
Suvashri Sasmal, Rakhi Gaur
- Professional Values *63*
- Professional Socialization: Integration of Professional Values with Personal Values *71*
- Professional Values in Nursing *77*
- Caring: Definition and Process *78*
- Compassion: Sympathy Versus Empathy and Altruism *82*
- Conscientiousness *86*
- Dedication/Devotion to Work *89*

- ❖ Respect for the Person-Human Dignity *91*
- ❖ Privacy and Confidentiality: Incidental Disclosure *93*
- ❖ Honesty and Integrity: Truth-Telling *96*
- ❖ Trust and Credibility: Fidelity and Loyalty *98*
- ❖ Advocacy *100*

Unit 3: Ethics and Bioethics

Chapter 5: Ethics and Bioethics — 107
Shiv Kumar Mudgal, Rakhi Gaur
- ❖ Meaning of Ethics, Morality, Bioethics *107*
- ❖ Ethical Principles *109*
- ❖ Application of Ethical Principles *109*

Chapter 6: Ethical Issues and Ethical Dilemma — 118
Rakhi Gaur, Shiv Kumar Mudgal
- ❖ Meaning of Ethical Dilemma *118*
- ❖ Conflict of Interest *119*
- ❖ Paternalism *120*
- ❖ Deception *121*
- ❖ Confidentiality and Privacy *122*
- ❖ Informed Consent and Refusal *124*
- ❖ Allocation of Scarce Health Resources *126*
- ❖ Conflicts Concerning New Technologies *127*
- ❖ Whistleblowing *128*
- ❖ Issues Related to Beginning of Life *130*
- ❖ Issues Related to End of Life *142*
- ❖ Issues Related to Psychiatric Care *151*

Chapter 7: Ethical Decision Making — 157
Jaison Joseph, Rakhi Gaur
- ❖ Ethical Decision-making in Nursing *157*
- ❖ Significance of Ethical Decision-making Process *157*
- ❖ The Process of Ethical Decision-making *158*
- ❖ Issues in Ethical Decision Making *162*
- ❖ Ethics Committee *163*

Chapter 8: Code of Ethics and Patient Rights — 170
Navjot Kaur, Shiv Kumar Mudgal
- ❖ Code of Ethics *170*
- ❖ Patient's Rights *179*

Index *191*

Syllabus

Professionalism, Professional Values and Ethics Including Bioethics

Placement: IV Semester

Theory: 1 Credit (20 hours)

Description: This course is designed to help students to develop an understanding of professionalism and demonstrate professional behavior in their workplace with ethics and professional values. Further the students will be able to identify ethical issues in nursing practice and participate effectively in ethical decision making along with health team members.

Competencies: On completion of this course, the students will be able to

- Describe profession and professionalism.
- Identify the challenges of professionalism.
- Maintain respectful communication and relationship with other health team members, patients and society.
- Demonstrate professional conduct.
- Describe various regulatory bodies and professional organizations related to nursing.
- Discuss the importance of professional values in patient care.
- Explain the professional values and demonstrate appropriate professional values in nursing practice.
- Demonstrate and reflect on the role and responsibilities in providing compassionate care in the healthcare setting.
- Demonstrate respect, human dignity and privacy and confidentiality to self, patients and their caregivers and other health team members.
- Advocate for patients' wellbeing, professional growth and advancing the profession.
- Identify ethical and bioethical concerns, issues and dilemmas in nursing and health care.
- Apply knowledge of ethics and bioethics in ethical decision making along with health team members.
- Protect and respect patient's rights.

COURSE OUTLINE

T – Theory, P – Practicum

Unit	Time (Hrs)	Learning Outcomes	Content	Teaching/ Learning Activities	Assessment Methods
I	5 (T)	Discuss nursing as a profession	**PROFESSIONALISM** **Profession** • Definition of profession • Criteria of a profession • Nursing as a profession	• Lecture cum Discussion	• Short answer • Essay • Objective type
		Describe the concepts and attributes of professionalism	**Professionalism** • Definition and characteristics of professionalism • Concepts, attributes and indicators of professionalism • *Challenges of professionalism*		
		Identify the challenges of professionalism	– Personal identity vs professional identity – Preservation of self-integrity: threat to integrity, Deceiving patient: withholding information and falsifying records – Communication and Relationship with team members: Respectful and open communication and relationship pertaining to relevant interests for ethical decision making – Relationship with patients and society	• Debate	
		Maintain respectful communication and relationship with other health team members, patients and society		• Role play	
		Demonstrate professional conduct	**Professional Conduct** Following ethical principles • Adhering to policies, rules and regulation of the institutions • Professional etiquettes and behaviors • Professional grooming: Uniform, Dress code • Professional boundaries: Professional relationship with the patients, caregivers and team members	• Case-based discussion	
		Respect and maintain professional boundaries between patients, colleagues and society			

Syllabus

Unit	Time (Hrs)	Learning Outcomes	Content	Teaching/ Learning Activities	Assessment Methods
		Describe the roles and responsibilities of regulatory bodies and professional organizations	**Regulatory Bodies and Professional Organizations: Roles and Responsibilities** • *Regulatory bodies*: Indian Nursing Council, State Nursing Council • *Professional Organizations*: Trained Nurses Association of India (TNAI), Student Nurses Association (SNA), Nurses League of Christian Medical Association of India, International Council of Nurses (ICN) and International Confederation of Midwives	• Lecture cum Discussion • Visit to INC, SNC, TNAI	• Visit reports
II	5 (T)	Discuss the importance of professional values Distinguish between personal values and professional values Demonstrate appropriate professional values in nursing practice	**PROFESSIONAL VALUES** • Values: Definition and characteristics of values • Value clarification • Personal and professional values • Professional socialization: Integration of professional values with personal values **Professional values in nursing** • Importance of professional values in nursing and health care • Caring: Definition, and process • Compassion: Sympathy Vs empathy, Altruism • Conscientiousness • Dedication/devotion to work • Respect for the person- Human dignity • Privacy and confidentiality: Incidental disclosure • Honesty and integrity: Truth telling • Trust and credibility: Fidelity, Loyalty • Advocacy: Advocacy for patients, work environment, nursing education and practice, and for advancing the profession	• Lecture cum Discussion • Value clarification exercise • Interactive learning • Story telling • Sharing experiences • Scenario-based discussion	• Short answer • Essay • Assessment of student's behavior with patients and families

Unit	Time (Hrs)	Learning Outcomes	Content	Teaching/ Learning Activities	Assessment Methods
III	10 (T)	Define ethics and bioethics	**ETHICS and BIOETHICS** Definitions: Ethics, Bioethics and Ethical Principles • Beneficence	• Lecture cum discussion • Group	• Short answer • Essay • Quiz • Reflective
		Explain ethical principles	• Non-maleficence: Patient safety, protecting patient from harm, Reporting errors	discussion with examples • Flipping/	diary • Case report • Attitude test • Assessment of
		Identify ethical concerns	• Justice: Treating each person as equal • Care without discrimination, equitable access to care and safety of the public • Autonomy: Respects patients' autonomy, Self-determination, Freedom of choice	self-directed learning • Role play • Story telling • Sharing experiences • Case-based Clinical discussion	assignment
		Ethical issues and dilemmas in health care	**Ethical issues and ethical dilemma: Common ethical problems** **Conflict of interest** • Paternalism • Deception • Privacy and confidentiality • Valid consent and refusal • Allocation of scarce nursing resources • Conflicts concerning new technologies • Whistle-blowing • *Beginning of life issues* − Abortion − Substance abuse	• Role modeling • Group exercise on ethical decision-making following steps on a given scenario • Assignment	
		Explain process of ethical decision making and apply knowledge of ethics and bioethics in making ethical decisions	− Fetal therapy − Selective deduction − Intrauterine treatment of fetal conditions − Mandated contraception − Fetal injury − Infertility treatment • *End of life issues* − End of life − Euthanasia − Do Not Resuscitate (DNR)		
		Explain code of ethics stipulated by ICN and INC	• *Issues related to psychiatric care* − Non compliance − Restrain and seclusion − Refuse to take food		

Unit	Time (Hrs)	Learning Outcomes	Content	Teaching/ Learning Activities	Assessment Methods
		Discuss the rights of the patients and families to make decisions about health care Protect and respect patients' rights	**Process of ethical decision making** • Assess the situation (collect information) • Identify the ethical problem • Identify the alternative decisions • Choose the solution to the ethical decision • Implement the decision • Evaluate the decision **Ethics committee: Roles and responsibilities** • Clinical decision making • Research • Code of Ethics • International Council of Nurses (ICN) • Indian Nursing Council **Patients' Bill of Rights-17 Patients' Rights (MoH&FW, GoI)** 1. Right to emergency medical care 2. Right to safety and quality care according to standards 3. Right to preserve dignity 4. Right to nondiscrimination 5. Right to privacy and confidentiality 6. Right to information 7. Right to records and reports 8. Right to informed consent 9. Right to second opinion 10. Right to patient education 11. Right to choose alternative treatment options if available 12. Right to choose source for obtaining medicines or tests 13. Right to proper referral and transfer, which is free from perverse commercial influences 14. Right to take discharge of patient or receive body of deceased from hospital		

Unit	Time (Hrs)	Learning Outcomes	Content	Teaching/ Learning Activities	Assessment Methods
			1. Right to information on the rates to be charged by the hospital for each type of service provided and facilities available on a prominent display board and a brochure 2. Right to protection for patients involved in clinical trials, biomedical and health research 3. Right to be heard and seek redressal		

UNIT 1

Professionals in Nursing

CHAPTER 1

Profession and Professionalism

T Johnsy Rani, R Beutlin

Learning Objectives

Upon completion of this chapter, the student should be able to:
- Define the profession
- Explain the criteria of a profession
- Describe nursing as a profession
- Define professionalism and its characteristics
- Explain the concepts, attributes, and indicators of professionalism
- Discuss the challenges of professionalism

■ PROFESSION

There are many educational courses one can opt after the school education, such as academic programs and professional programs. The academic programs focus more on the theoretical aspects and are referred to as liberal courses which include Bachelor of Arts (BA), Bachelor of Commerce (BCom), etc. On the contrary, professional programs, such as Medicine (Bachelor of Medicine and Bachelor of Surgery), Engineering (Bachelor of Engineering), Nursing (Bachelor of Science in Nursing) and Paramedical courses (Physiotherapy, Occupational therapy, Laboratory technology, etc.) are aimed at the cultivation of practical skills that enables a person to work in a particular field with specific skills. The professional courses prepare specialized experts in a specific field through intensive training that can be applied to a variety of job-related situations.

Meaning

The term "profession" is derived from the English word "profess" which means 'to proclaim something publicly'. A profession is a job, occupation, or vocation in which an individual work and has received formal training. Professions are those occupations possessing a particular combination of characteristics generally considered to be expertise, autonomic, committed, and responsible.

A profession is an occupation based on specialized intellectual study and training, the purpose of which is to supply skilled services.

Definitions

"An occupation whose core element is work based upon the mastery of a complex body of knowledge and skills. It is a vocation in which knowledge of some department of science or learning or the practice of an art founded upon it is used in the service of others."
—**Sylvia RC, 2010**

"Profession is any type of work that needs special training or a particular skill, often one that is respected because it involves a high level of education." —**Cambridge Dictionary**

"Profession is a chosen, paid, occupation that requires a prolonged training and formal qualification." —**Oxford Dictionary**

"An occupation in which an individual uses an intellectual skill based on an established body of knowledge and practice to provide a specialized service in a defined area, exercising independent judgement following a code of ethics and in the public interest."
—**The UK Inter-professional Group**

In nutshell, a profession can be viewed as an occupation with specialized study and training bounded by ethical standards to serve mankind.

Differences between Occupation and Profession

Although the terms "occupation" and "profession" are sometimes used interchangeably, the meanings of these terms in a more general sense are very different. Profession is an occupation, but all occupations are not professions. Understanding these differences helps to easily identify and distinguish between an occupation and profession. Refer **Table 1.1** for differences between an occupation and profession.

TABLE 1.1: Differences between occupation and profession.

Aspects of comparison	Occupation	Profession
Meaning	Occupation refers to a person's regular activity that he or she does to earn a living	A profession is an occupation that needs a high level of knowledge and skill in a particular sector
Code of conduct	No	Yes
Formal training	It is not mandatory	It is essential
Regulated by statute	No	Yes
Values, beliefs, and ethics	Not considered as the most essential component of training	Considered as an essential component of training

Characteristics of a Profession

Characteristics refer to features that stand unique and differentiate from common things. The main characteristics of a profession are illustrated in **Figure 1.1**.

- ❖ **Specialized body of knowledge:** Professionals render specialized services based on theory, knowledge, and skills that are most often peculiar to their profession. This provides the framework for the practice.
- ❖ **Professional standards and code of ethics:** A profession is based on a general body of core values and standards set by the concerned regulatory bodies of the profession.
- ❖ **Set of skills for specific services:** A profession stands to provide specialized services based on a set of skills distinct to that profession. Therefore, each profession is entrusted with great responsibilities and obligations toward society.
- ❖ **Standardized formal education:** Every profession is based on a standardized formal education controlled by various regulatory bodies. This helps in the preparation of competent members with

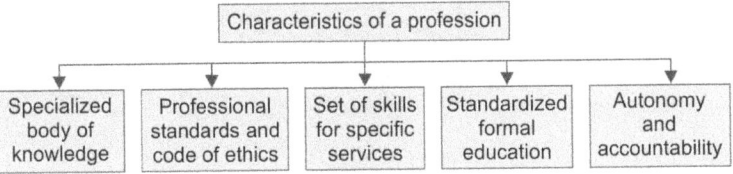

Fig. 1.1: Characteristics of a profession.

practical experience in the protected environment that is typically required for a particular profession.

❖ **Autonomy and accountability:** Members of a profession have the freedom for making decisions and are answerable for their actions while rendering their services.

CRITERIA OF A PROFESSION

Criteria are the principles or standards for evaluating a profession. Many authors have explained the criteria of the profession in different ways. Some of the major criteria which explain a profession are listed below:

According to Flexner (1915)

Abraham Flexner has stated six criteria for a profession **(Fig. 1.2)**:

1. A profession is based on *intellectual* activities (as opposed to physical) and is accompanied by a high degree of individual responsibility.
2. The practice of a profession is founded on a *body of knowledge* that may be learned and is expanded and improved via research.
3. In addition to focusing on theory, the professional activities emphasize *practical* application.

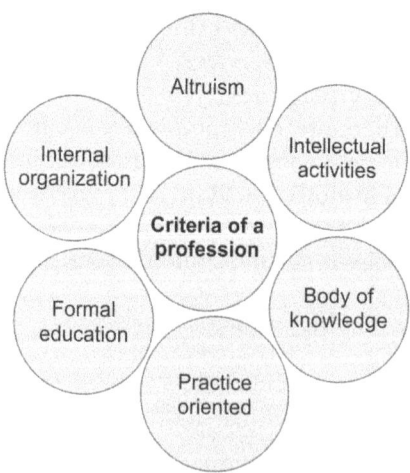

Fig. 1.2: Flexner's criteria of a profession.

4. Techniques of a profession are taught through a highly specialized process of *formal education*.
5. The profession has a well-developed group consciousness and a robust *internal organizational structure* of members.
6. Practitioners in the profession are driven by *altruism* (a willingness to serve others) and are interested in public concerns.

According to Bixler and Bixler (1945)

The following are considered as the criteria for a profession **(Fig. 1.3)**:

- ❖ **Intellectual and has body of knowledge:** The members practicing in the profession utilizes highly specialized knowledge and technical skill for their practice. The members of the profession are trained in all domains – cognitive, affective, and psychomotor to develop competency.
- ❖ **Essential services:** The services provided by a profession should be ultimately aimed at providing service to human and social welfare. The services are necessary for survival and they cannot be substituted by others.
- ❖ **Continuous professional growth:** The profession should offer its members organized opportunities for continued professional growth. It can be done through continuing education, on-job training, seminars, workshops, conference, etc.

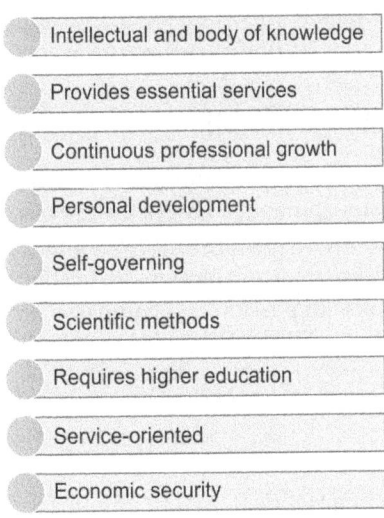

Fig. 1.3: Bixler's criteria for profession.

- **Personal development:** Professionals are encouraged to work with the confidence and implement new ideas and procedures. They have the right to question and assess what is being done. Professionals have a lot of opportunities to improve and develop their practice because of this freedom.
- **Self-governing:** A genuine profession will give and cultivate leadership abilities among its members. They facilitate the establishment of policies and norms for professional activities.
- **Scientific:** A professional person's education is built on a foundation of scientific knowledge. Every profession has its own body of knowledge from which the members utilize the knowledge for their routine professional practice. A genuine profession will continue to research while also utilizing the developing amount of information and the expertise of its practitioners.
- **Requires higher education:** A professional person should be educated in a higher educational institution, i.e., colleges that are regulated by the universities. Apart from it, higher qualifications and specialization can be done to improve professional practice.
- **Service-oriented:** Members of the profession are supposed to spend most of their energy on it for the rest of their lives.
- **Economic security:** A profession provides economic security to its members for their service. Economic security means having an adequate amount of money to meet the daily expenses without any interruption which is important for an individual. This economic security is an asset during retirement time as well.

NURSING AS A PROFESSION

The word "nurse" is derived from the Latin word "nutire" which means "to nurture or foster someone". Therefore, the nursing profession is ideal for someone who is looking to serve humanity. It is said to be a very noble profession because it requires dedication and commitment to care for patients with passion and compassion. Apart from these, nursing has indeed a very profitable career and has international scope as well.

Definition

According to Virginia Henderson, "the unique function of the nurse is to assist the individual, sick or well, in the performance of those activities contributing to health or its recovery (or to peaceful death) that he/she would perform unaided if he had the necessary strength, will or knowledge, and to do this in such a way as to help him gain independence as rapidly as possible."

Qualities of a Nurse

There are certain fundamental qualities that a nurse must possess while rendering their service in their professional areas which are listed below **(Fig. 1.4)**:

- **Caring:** Quality of caring makes a difference in patients. A nurse showing a natural tendency to truly care about how their patients feel will have a significant impact on their success in the nursing field, which makes caring a key indicator of a nurse's success.
- **Communication skills:** Communication is sharing of information. To be a successful healthcare provider nurses need exceptional communication ability. The capacity of a nurse to communicate effectively is crucial. A nurse's ability to communicate successfully with other nurses, and other health team members across different units, patients, and their families is vital to their job.

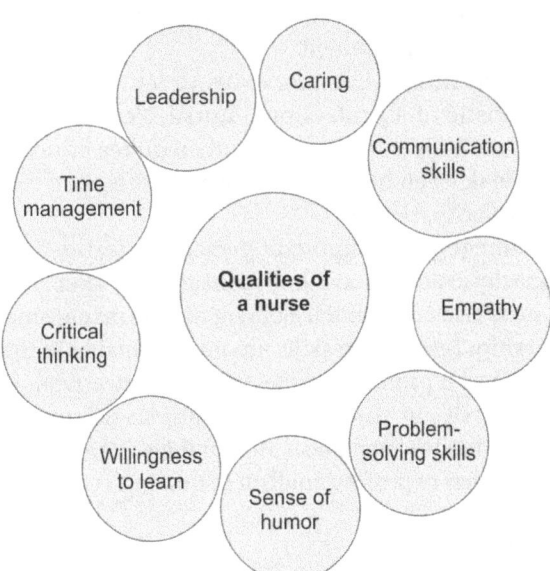

Fig. 1.4: Qualities of a nurse.

- **Empathy:** A competent nurse empathizes with each patient and makes an honest attempt to put oneself in the shoes of their patients. Empathetic nurses are more inclined to regard their patient as "person", focusing on a person-centered approach to care rather than strictly following protocol. An empathetic nurse can enhance the treatment experience of their patients dramatically.
- **Problem-solving skills:** Problem-solving skills are essential to nursing, as nurses generally spend most of their time with patients. Nurses are often responsible for much of the decision-making related to their care. Even small decisions can have major impacts on outcomes.
- **Sense of humor:** Possessing a strong sense of humor aids in creating positivity in fellow professional colleagues, patients, and their families. Patients and their families are extremely grateful for any efforts to offer brightness, particularly during stressful periods.
- **Willingness to learn:** Development in educational methodologies (e.g., collaborative training, individualized learning, etc.) may aid in the creation of successful learning environments, but a competent nurse must have an innate desire to learn to be genuinely effective. Nurses of all ages, from young graduates to seasoned experts, can benefit from this critical skills in every phases of their employment.
- **Critical thinking:** A strong drive to learn is an important characteristic of a professional nurse. Nevertheless, putting knowledge into practice successfully requires critical thinking. While this skill can be developed over time, it often comes more readily with experience.
- **Time management:** Important personality feature for nurses is the capacity to adopt good time management. Allocating time for self-care is also an essential element of time management.
- **Leadership:** Leadership skills are more valuable in the nursing profession as it promotes professional advancement. Exercising leadership skills in any role or level shows a willingness to grow and adapt at one's own pace. Mentorships from nursing leaders are the sources of professionalism in nursing.

■ **Critical Thinking**
Does cultural diversity affect the quality of nurses?

Roles and Responsibilities of a Nurse

One of the most important aspects of professional nursing practice in the art of nursing is to assist individuals, families, and communities. The following are the essential roles entrusted to professionals in the nursing profession **(Fig. 1.5)**:

* **Caregiver:** It encompasses all efforts aimed at assisting the client physically and psychologically while maintaining his or her dignity. This includes complete or partial care for the clients based on their ability to perform the activities of daily living. The nurse provides educational and supportive care to help the clients to achieve their optimum level of health and wellness and delegates the responsibilities to the caregivers.
* **Teacher:** As a teacher, the nurse helps the clients to learn about their health and health care practices that they need to perform to restore or maintain their health. The nurse assesses the client's learning needs and readiness to learn, sets specific learning goals following the priorities, and utilizes various teaching strategies.
* **Communicator:** Effective communication is an integral factor in nursing care. To address the client's health care needs, the nurse must be able to communicate effectively and properly. Nurses communicate with clients and assist family members and community members. Nurses who play the job of communicator recognize clients' problems and then communicate them to other

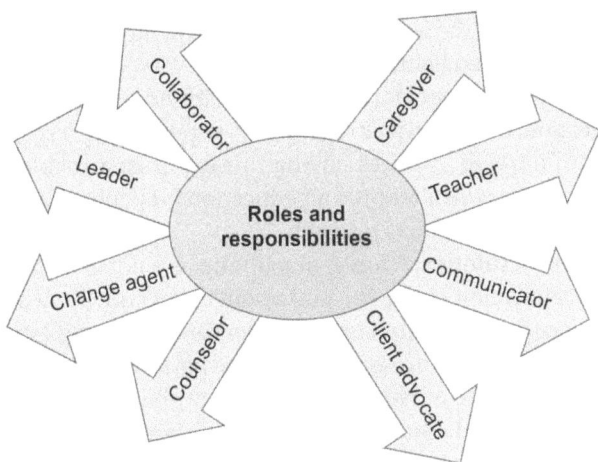

Fig. 1.5: Roles and responsibilities of a nurse.

professionals of the health team verbally or in writing. The quality of a nurse's communication is an important factor in nursing care.
- ❖ **Client advocate:** As a client advocate, a nurse acts to protect the client. Nurses assist clients in exercising their rights and help them speak up for themselves.
- ❖ **Counselor:** Counseling is the process of helping a client to recognize and cope with psychological or social problems, develop interpersonal relationships, and promote growth. A nurse counsels and helps the person to develop new attitudes, and behaviors encouraging the client to look at alternative behavior and recognize the choices.
- ❖ **Change agent:** The nurse acts as a change agent when assisting clients to make modifications in the behaviors.
- ❖ **Leader:** A leader influences others to work for accomplishing a specific goal. A nurse takes up the leader's role, by performing in an assertive and self-confident manner for bringing effective change and functioning in professional activities.
- ❖ **Collaborator:** A nurse acts as a collaborator with effective use of skill in organization, communication, and advocacy to facilitate the functions of all health team members as they provide patient care.

Expanded Educational and Career Roles of Nurses

The nurse performs certain advanced roles based on the qualification and regulations of the governing body. Some of the extended roles of the nurses are listed below:
- ❖ **Clinical nurse specialist:** A nurse with an advanced degree, education, or expertise is regarded as a specialist in a specialized area of nursing. A nurse having this expertise provides direct patient care, consultation, and education for patient, family, and staff and also conducts research.
- ❖ **Nurse practitioner:** A nurse practitioner is a nurse who attained the qualification of a nurse practitioner program. Their scope of practice (power granted to a provider) and privileges (spectrum of health facilities) are governed by the laws of the state in which they work. Some nurse practitioners may practice in hospitals or clinics without the supervision of a physician. Others collaborate with doctors as part of a multidisciplinary health care team.

- ❖ **Nurse midwife:** A nurse who accomplishes a program in midwifery provides prenatal and postnatal care to women with uncomplicated pregnancies and delivers their babies.
- ❖ **Nurse educator:** A nurse with an advanced degree is involved in educational activities in academic or clinical settings to impart theoretical and practical information.
- ❖ **Nurse administrator:** A nurse is responsible for the management and administration of resources and staff in providing patient care at various levels of management in health care settings.
- ❖ **Nurse researcher:** Nurse researcher is the one who has an advanced degree and who conduct research for the improvement of nursing practice and education.
- ❖ **Nurse entrepreneur:** A nurse entrepreneur is a nurse usually with an advanced degree who manages a clinic or a health-related business, conduct research, provides education, or serves as an advisor or consultant to institutions, political agencies, or businesses.
- ❖ **Forensic nurse:** Individuals who are victims or perpetrators of trauma receive specialized care from forensic nurses. Forensic nurses understand the legal system and are skilled at identifying, evaluating, and documenting injuries.
- ❖ **Nurse informatics:** Nurse informatics is nursing specialists that integrate their nursing expertise with their understanding of computer science. They work with data gathering, organizing, and interpreting to improve the efficiency and quality of patient care. They work in a variety of contexts, including insurance companies, hospitals, and consulting organizations.

CHARACTERISTICS OF THE NURSING PROFESSION

Certain characteristics make nursing a unique profession as compared to other professions which are listed below **(Fig. 1.6)**:
- ❖ **Nursing is caring:** Caring is the dynamic core and most vital quality in nursing. Caring is essential in the nursing profession because it helps with the healing process. It is a way for nurses to show empathy and compassion towards their patients. Being kind is the essential quality that must be possessed by the nurse through which the patients can understand caring.

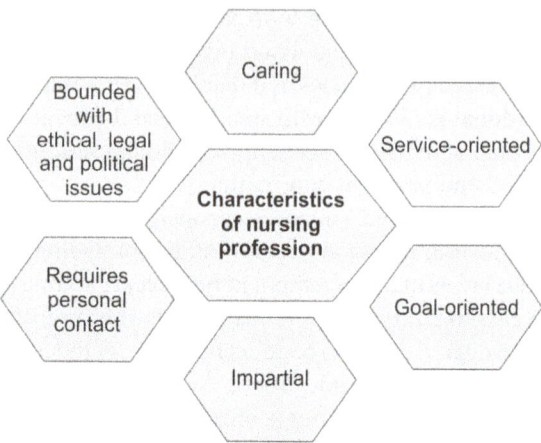

Fig. 1.6: Characteristics of the nursing profession.

- ❖ **Nursing is service-oriented:** Nursing considers persons as physiological, psychological, and sociological beings. Nursing is a call to service focusing on the preventive, promotive, curative, and rehabilitative aspects of the person as a whole. Nursing services are rendered with dedication and commitment.
- ❖ **Nursing is goal-oriented:** Nursing is intended to help people achieve their personal, family, community, and universal healthcare goals in the most effective way possible. Nurses formulate specific and realistic goals that can be measured in real-time to ensure patient progress within a specified time frame.
- ❖ **Nursing is impartial:** Nursing is dedicated to provide individualized care to all people, regardless of race, religion, economic or social position. All persons are treated with utmost respect and dignity without any discrimination.
- ❖ **Nursing requires personal contact:** Nursing involves close personal contact with the recipient of care, such as patients, families, and communities. Care and cure coordinated concept is applied in providing the care.
- ❖ **Nursing is bounded by ethical, legal, and political issues:** Ethical, legal, and political issues related to nursing are an important area of concern when dealing with the human being. In these difficulties, the professional code of ethics in nursing serves as a set of norms for nurses' behaviour and provides general recommendations for nursing actions.

Criteria of the Nursing Profession

Nursing is considered the "youngest of the professions". Nursing has been merged as a learned profession which is a science and an art. Nursing is a science, which requires a sound type of education and a thorough knowledge of human behavior. Nursing is an art in which skills are developed by practice. In addition to scientific knowledge and skills, desirable attitudes are necessary for nursing. Therefore, the basic requirements for a nurse are the knowledge of nursing science (head), the desire to nurse, the spirit of nursing (heart), and the attitude and the skill of nursing (hand).

Nursing fulfills most of the criteria of a profession. The following are the criteria that fulfill nursing as a profession:

- **Essential services:** Nursing services are critical to mankind and the well-being of society. Nursing is a service to the well-being of individuals and society as a whole. Nursing fosters the preservation and recovery of individuals', groups', and communities' health. The prime objective of the nursing profession is to help others to achieve the best level of well-being in which they are competent. Caring means nurturing and helping others and it is the basic component of professional nursing.
- **Body of knowledge:** There is a special body of knowledge, which is continually enlarged through research in nursing. In the past, nursing was based on principles borrowed from the physical and social sciences and other disciplines. Today, however, there is a body of knowledge for nursing. Currently, the nursing profession relies more on research as a basis for practice than on task orientation, intuition, or trial and error.
- **Intellectual activities:** The nursing services incorporate intellectual activities. Nursing has developed and refined its unique approach to the practice called the nursing process. The nursing process is essentially a cognitive (mental) activity that requires both critical and creative thinking and serves as the basis for providing nursing care. Accountability is the process in which individuals are answerable for their actions and have the obligation to act. Nurses are accountable to themselves, clients and their families, and the general public.
- **Formal higher education:** Practitioners in nursing are educated in institutions of higher learning. After the formal basic qualification

in nursing, nurses continue their higher education as post-graduation and doctoral programs in colleges and universities.

- ❖ **Autonomy:** Practitioners in nursing are relatively independent and control their policies and activities. Autonomy or control over one's practice is another controversial area for nursing. While many nursing actions are independent, the nurse practice acts vary according to country and across the globe.
- ❖ **Altruism:** Altruism means being selfless and concern for the well-being of others. Nursing professionals render their service to help others and see their work as an important part of their lives.
- ❖ **Code of ethics:** A code of ethics governs the decisions and actions of nursing professionals. An ethical code does not describe how an individual should act in a specific situation; rather, it provides professional standards and a framework for decision-making. The trust placed in the nursing profession by the public requires that the nurses must act with integrity. To aid them in doing so, both the International Council of Nurses (ICN) and the Indian Nursing Council (INC) have developed codes of nursing ethics that establish, promote, and refine standards of practice.
- ❖ **Professional associations:** The professional associations promote and support high standards of nursing practice. A variety of professional associations in nursing have been established to advance the profession. The goal of which is to create high standards of nursing practice, promote the professional and educational advancement of nurses, and promote the welfare of nurses to improve nursing care for all individuals. The organizations advocate for nursing concerns in general and serve as the official voice of nursing. In India, 'The Trained Nurses' Association of India' (TNAI) and the State Government Nurses Association are some of the professional associations in nursing.

PROFESSIONALISM

Nursing has changed from a mere job into a profession through the recent increase in professional independence with the development of definitions for roles and performances. Professionalism has become one of the important basis in nursing due to the gradual development of educational standards and professional advancement. Nurses are the largest group of healthcare workers, and their professional abilities play a critical part in the development of a functional healthcare system. It encompasses the use of knowledge and abilities, performance of routine tasks, leadership, self-discipline, professional dedication, and social ideals.

Meaning

Professionalism is not the job or the task the professional does, but it is the way of doing the job or the task.

Professionalism is a set of activities, tasks, and nurse's duties carried out by registered nurses, at any time whenever it is required keeping the person's health as their priority.

Professionalism in nursing means embodying core values of integrity, responsibility, advocacy, and accountability.

Professionalism is a practice that can benefit everyone in the healthcare setting, including patients, caregivers, co-workers, and self.

Definitions

Professionalism is defined as "the conceptualization of obligations, attributes, interactions, attitudes and role behaviors required of professionals in relation to individual clients and society as a whole."
—**Richard LC, 2000**

Professionalism is defined as "the consistent demonstration of core values evidenced by nurses working with other professionals to achieve optimal health and wellness outcomes in patients, families, and communities by wisely applying principles of altruism, excellence, caring, ethics, respect, communication, and accountability."
—**American Association of Colleges of Nursing, 2008**

Professionalism is defined as "the personally held beliefs of a professional about their conduct as a member of a profession. It is often linked to upholding of the principles, laws, ethics, and conventions of a profession in the form of a code of practice."
—**Australian Council of Professions, 2003**

Characteristics of Professionalism

Professionalism is characterized by autonomous evidence-based decision-making by members of occupation who share the same values and education. It demonstrates an unwavering commitment to the vocation and the willingness to continuously deliver the highest-quality care to patients. It is realized through purposeful relationships and underpinned by environments that facilitate professional practice. The characteristics of professionalism in nursing are described below (**Fig. 1.7**):

- ❖ **Self-regulation:** It includes the control of professional activities and practices through quality assurance approaches, such as licensure, accreditation, etc. In India, a national independent regulating organization, the Indian Nursing Council, monitors and regulates the nursing profession in conjunction with each autonomous state nursing council. The Indian Nursing Council manages a nationwide database registry. In general, state nursing councils have the authority to approve nursing education programs, in collaboration with the Indian Nursing Council. Each state nursing council in India is responsible for the registration, licensing, and disciplining of nursing professionals. State nursing councils have the authority to implement nursing laws and regulations and to regulate for the protection of the public.
- ❖ **Self-determination:** The nursing profession is still striving to determine its own choices, role on the health care team, and future professional destiny. Nurses themselves are the best personnel to understand the demands of their profession and are therefore entitled to devise strategies for its future direction. Nurses assert themselves and turn increasingly to collective bargaining for negotiating professional issues.

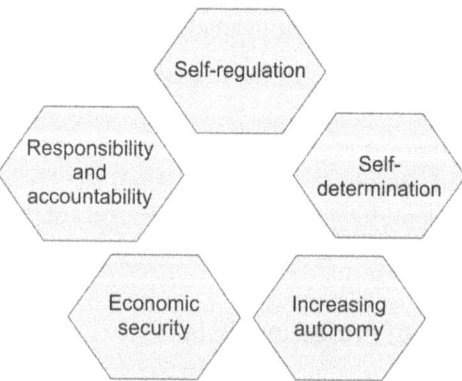

Fig. 1.7: Characteristics of professionalism.

- **Responsibility and accountability:** Currently, nurses are involved in more complex patient care activities and the responsibilities are shifted from traditional nursing care to independent nursing practice. As a result of the increased freedom in practice, the responsibility for nursing actions is further moved to accountability. Nurses have to achieve a balance between their responsibility and accountability to safeguard the public and concern for their welfare.
- **Increasing autonomy:** Autonomy refers to the freedom to practice while rendering service among the members of a profession. Nursing utilizes the existing body of knowledge, code of ethics, and professional conduct while making decisions related to the various aspects of patient care activities.
- **Economic security:** Economic gains are the most observable and socially understandable needs sought by the nursing profession. Though the economic picture for nurses has changed radically in the past two decades, economic security has still become a top priority in the nursing profession. The low wages and poor working conditions are the major constraints faced by the nurses due to disparities in the legislation in the various employment setting.

■ **Critical Thinking**
1. What is the best title for nursing in the context of professionalism?
2. What are the major characteristics that make nursing distinct from other disciplines in the health care system?

Attributes of Professionalism

Professionalism means the act of behaving in a manner that is expected by a given profession. The attributes or the expected fundamental qualities of nursing professionals were initially advocated by Florence Nightingale. They included patient care, cleanliness, and management, to achieve a higher degree of professionalism and standards. The following are the essential attributes or fundamental features of professionalism in the context of nursing (**Fig. 1.8**):

- **Knowledge:** The knowledge regarding the various aspects of nursing is critical for the nurse while performing nursing practice. The particular theoretical idea helps the nurse to apply that knowledge which becomes a rationale for professional activities and practice.

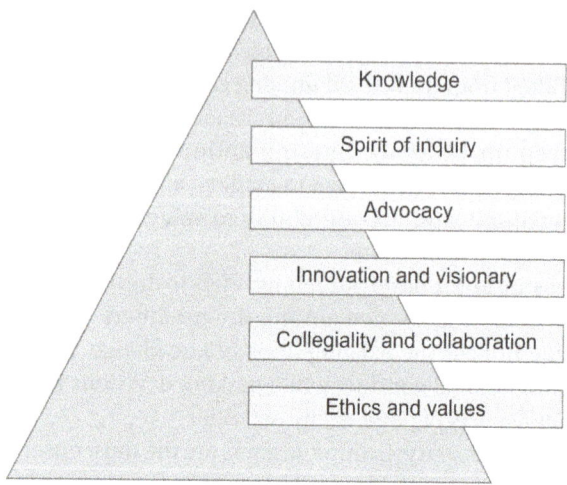

Fig. 1.8: Attributes of professionalism.

- ❖ **Spirit of inquiry:** One of the distinctive characteristics of a professional nurse would be the inquisitive nature or the curiosity for learning. To improve the quality of patient care, nurses exhibit this characteristic by making observations, creating questions, and collecting and analyzing data. It is necessary to examine critically and think creatively to bolster one's knowledge base to make educated healthcare decisions. A strong commitment and genuine interest are of pivotal importance to explore new knowledge.
- ❖ **Advocacy:** One of the essential ideas of professional nursing practice is advocacy, which demands nurses empower patients to make informed decisions by defending their rights, interests, and beliefs. Nurses can participate in the development of health policies that enhance the work environment and patient outcomes. In addition to recognizing and respecting the scope of practice of other healthcare professionals, nurses can identify and develop successful working relationships with important stakeholders to enhance client autonomy. However, lack of support from healthcare team members is considered a significant barrier to patient advocacy.
- ❖ **Innovation and visionary:** Innovation and vision refer to the introduction of novel concepts or imaginative insights to enhance patient care and achieve favorable outcomes.

Innovative nursing has a favorable effect on professional practice since it seeks to enhance job satisfaction and care quality. It allows nurses to participate in quality improvement projects and think imaginatively. By challenging the established conditions and recognizing chances that improve nursing practice, nurses can demonstrate their inventiveness. Using reflective practice and curiosity, the nurse promotes innovation to improve the quality of the health care setting.

- **Collegiality and collaboration:** Professionalism entails forming collaborative relationships with other healthcare providers and displaying collegiality. They are seen as important predictors of positive patient outcomes, enhanced teamwork, job satisfaction, effective nurse-physician relationships, autonomy, and quality care. By having a clear awareness of their scope of practice and recognizing and respecting the roles of other health care team members, nurses can foster collegiality and collaboration.
- **Ethics and values:** Professionalism in nursing can be achieved by providing safe, competent, and ethical nursing care. The nursing code of ethics encourages nurses to be accountable and professional. Knowing that nursing practice has an ethical dimension might help nurses create their professional identity. Nurses can use a variety of tools when making decisions to address ethical challenges in practice.

Concepts and Indicators of Professionalism in Nursing

Professionalism in nursing means providing top-quality care to patients, while also upholding the values of accountability, respect, and integrity.

Miller's Wheel of Professionalism in Nursing

Miller's Wheel of Professionalism in Nursing provides a framework for discussion of professional concepts in nursing. Barbara Kemp Miller created the "Wheel of Professionalism in Nursing" model in 1984 to study the concept of professionalism. The model was created in response to the need for nurses to be able to recognize the features and behaviors that characterize nursing professionalism. The model is represented as a wheel with hub and spokes. The hub represents essential qualities, while the spokes reflect supportive behaviors.

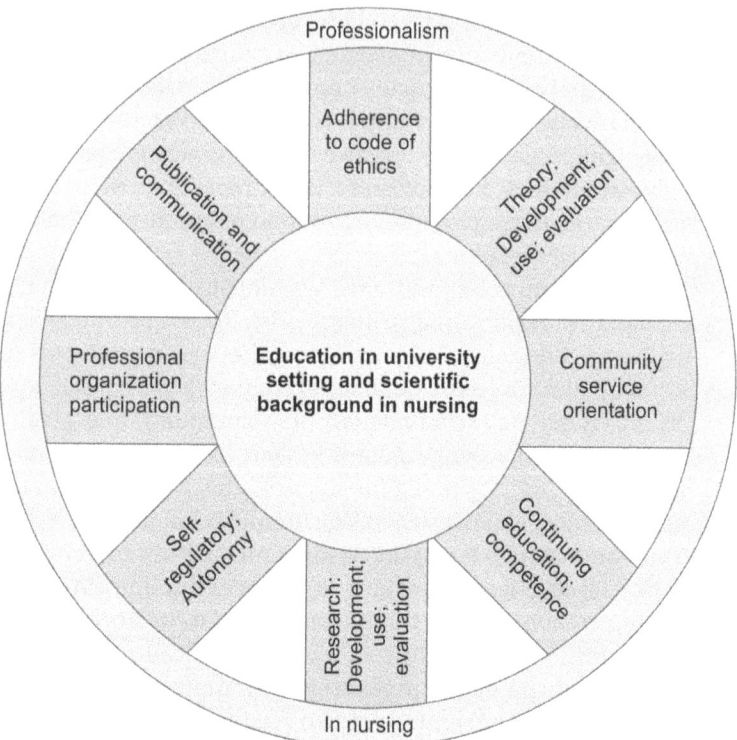

Fig. 1.9: Concepts of professionalism in nursing.

Professionalism—Core concepts: Two essential elements of nursing professionalism are represented by the hub or center of the wheel. Formal standardized education in an academic setting and a scientific background of knowledge are considered core concepts for establishing professionalism in nursing **(Fig. 1.9)**.

Professionalism—Indicators:- The spokes of the wheel depict the behaviors or indicators of professionalism which are listed below:

- ❖ **Adherence to the code of ethics:** The code of ethics acts as a guide and represents the symbol of professionalism. Professionalism necessitates adherence to the code of ethics for nurses and specifies the nursing profession's principles and beliefs. The nurses' code of ethics is seen as a significant instrument that enables nurses to practice ethically when dealing with ethical dilemmas in their nursing practice. In India, the code of ethics and code of professional conduct for nurses were formulated and enforced by the Indian nursing council and state nursing council.

- ❖ **Theory development and utilization:** A functional element of professionalism includes the development and utilization of theories relevant to the nursing profession. The evaluation of theories and integration of its findings into routine clinical practices serve as an indicator of professionalism in the nursing profession.
- ❖ **Community service:** Community service and public education are considered a basic indicators of professionalism in nursing. One of the most important aspects of professional nursing practice is the promotion of public health and well-being by assisting individuals, families, and communities. Nurses are dedicated to help patients, families, and communities by providing outreach services to preserve their health.
- ❖ **Competence and continuing education:** Professional competency has been proposed as a reflection of professionalism in nursing. Professional competency includes the combination of skills, knowledge, attitudes, values, and abilities that bring about effective or high performance in occupational and professional positions. Nurses must participate in continuing professional development to keep informed with developments in the healthcare profession. Nurses must learn new knowledge and skills to practice safely in new and expanded responsibilities.
- ❖ **Research development:** A sound understanding and participation in research help to understand and overcome the boundaries and limitations of nursing practice. The involvement of nurses in evidence-based research itself is an indicator of professionalism as it promotes inter-professional collaboration and dignity within and outside the profession.
- ❖ **Self-regulation and autonomy:** Nursing is a self-regulated profession in which professionals practice in a safe, competent, and ethical manner. The regulation of the nursing profession in India is achieved through the self-regulatory mechanisms of INC and state nursing council in the form of professional registration, license, etc. Autonomy or independence in nursing refers to the freedom to make judgements and use clinical decisions within the scope of standards of practice. Development and implementation

of effective patient care practices and assuming advanced practice roles such as nurse practitioner are ways of demonstrating autonomy in the nursing profession.

- ❖ **Participation in the professional organization:** Professionalism also necessitates participation in numerous professional organizations. Various nursing professional organizations (e.g., TNAI) are committed to maintaining self-regulation and control with an emphasis on public safety. Participation in professional organizations helps promotes a creative work atmosphere as it promotes professional affiliations and morale.
- ❖ **Publication and communication:** Publication and communication of the various perspectives of nursing is an additional professional behavior demonstrating professionalism. Writing for publication in nursing forms a primary source of the nursing literature. Communication of findings helps in the development of a structural or scientific base for the nursing profession. Reflecting critically and disseminating judiciously on the standards and effectiveness of practice forms the essence of professional activity in nursing.

■ CHALLENGES OF PROFESSIONALISM

Various factors might be challenging for the various dimensions of professionalism. Some of the factors that affect professional knowledge, professional competence, and professional commitment are described below.

I. Personal Identity vs. Professional Identity

Personal identity	*Professional identity*
Personal identity is considered as the totality of values, attitudes, memories, and aspirations that are unique to an individual. This reflects how one sees own self or relationship with self. These are the meanings that individuals hold for themselves to represent a unique biological entity	Professional identity is viewed as the attitudes, values, knowledge, beliefs, and skills shared with others within a professional group. It is a sense of identity in relationship with the profession in the form of achievements, such as publications, distinguished contributions, etc. It reflects the degree to which an individual identifies with his or her professional group

Contd...

Contd...

Challenges of professionalism: Professional identity

- **Gender:** Although gender was not identified as a criterion for professionalism, it plays a major role in perceiving professional identity in nursing. Traditionally, nursing was considered as a profession for women, therefore, there is a wide discrepancy exists in the professional identity of men in the profession in the form of job opportunities, job areas, and professional advancement.
- **Education:** The difference in the educational processes in nursing is a challenge to achieve a professional status of identity. Educational diversity within nursing resulted in the quality of education and training which has slowed the progress toward acceptance of the professional practice. In addition, the quality of nurse educators, availability of facilities, and demographic factors have a crucial role to determine the steady development of nursing as a profession.
- **Historical influences:** At the personal level, the nurse might be striving for collaboration and competition with other health personnel with whom they work. However, due to the perceived professional conflicts or social stigma, the nurses may not be able to express their unique knowledge, experience, and skills to exercise the experience of professional autonomy within the health care profession.
- **Role confusion:** Despite the achievement of higher education in nursing, the nurses often perceive a lack of recognition regarding the implication of their work. The influence of lobbying and unmet expectations as per their professional identity might result in a great deal of ambivalence toward the nursing profession.

Strategies to promote a professional identity

- Create a personal nursing philosophy to serve as a framework for practice.
- Become actively involved in professional nursing associations.
- Continuous striving for professional advancement through continuing education.
- Creating a professional image through academic success, publication, work experience, and verbal and nonverbal communication abilities.

The formation of a professional identity involves the acquisition of knowledge, competencies, attitudes, and values.

II. Preservation of Self-integrity

The trait of being fair and honest, and possessing strong moral principles are considered as characteristics of integrity. In nursing, integrity is concerned with the behaviors that promote trustworthiness in the patient and their family members.

Threats to Self-integrity

Threats to self-integrity in nursing include requests to deceive a patient, withhold information, or falsify records, as well as verbal abuse from patients or coworkers. A threat to integrity is in direct violation of the code of ethics or acting in a way beyond professional boundaries. Nurses have a responsibility to uphold their personal and professional ideals without compromising their self-respect.

Deceiving Patient: Withholding Information and Falsifying Records

Withholding Information

The treatment-related information must be communicated to the patients based on their choices and ability of understanding. Withholding of information is the intentional omission of concealing the information from the patient. However, sometimes it would be unintentional, which makes it difficult to evaluate morally. Truthful and open communication is essential for trust in the nurse-client relationship and respect for autonomy. Withholding relevant medical information from patients creates tension between the need to promote patient welfare and the obligation to protect patient autonomy. Withholding information without the patient's knowledge or agreement is unethical, except in emergency instances where a patient is incapable of making an informed decision. When information has been withheld in such circumstances, the nurse must provide that information once the emergency has been resolved.

Strategies to Overcome the Challenges Related to Disclosing or Withholding Information

- ❖ Assess the patient preferences regarding communication of medical information, preferably before the information becomes available.
- ❖ Accept the patient's rights of receiving or withholding information from himself or the nominated representative.
- ❖ Determine the client's ability level and reveal information to fulfill the patient's demands and expectations while respecting the individual's preferences.
- ❖ Any decision to withhold medically contraindicated information must be made in consultation with the patient's family and other members of the health care team after weighing the relative advantages and risks of postponing disclosure.
- ❖ Keep a close observation of the patient and provide complete disclosure when the patient can determine whether or not to access the information.

Falsifying Records

A long-standing, essential principle of nursing documentation is that it would be truthful and accurate. Making a false statement on any document with the intent to defame the patient or their primary providers are known as document falsification. Document or record falsification also includes unauthorized alteration or transmitting such documents to another person. The document in which falsification is commonly reported are patient care plans, medication administration records, patient treatment records, patients' vital signs records, etc.

Importance of Self-integrity in Nursing Practice

One of the most crucial things a nurse can do for herself, her patients, and her team is to practice self-integrity. The practice of self-integrity in nursing helps to promote trustworthiness and dependability among the health team members and patients and their caregivers. The practice of self-integrity in nursing also helps to enhance patient outcomes.

Strategies to Demonstrate Self-integrity in Nursing Practice

One of the most effective strategies to develop solid nurse-patient and professional relationships is to act with the highest levels of integrity. Maintaining integrity as a nurse means having a core set of principles and demonstrating them in all professional practices. Some of the strategies to demonstrate self-integrity in nursing practice are described below:

- **Be honest:** Integrity in nursing practice means being honest. The nurse can provide the truly granted care while being truthful.
- **Behaving respectfully:** Patients, regardless of their physical or mental ability or cultural background, should be treated with respect. It exhibits strong professional and personal integrity to treat everyone with the same regard and consideration.
- **Being accountable:** Being accountable in own actions is one of the best ways of demonstrating self-integrity.
- **Acknowledging others:** Recognizing the efforts of peers and patients is one of the methods to practice self-integrity in nursing. It further improves professional and patient outcomes as it upholds self-esteem.

- ❖ **Adherence to rules and regulations:** Adhering to the policies fosters a professional environment, which helps to maintain self-integrity.
- ❖ **Offering help:** Offering self for assisting others is great morale of conduct in nursing.
- ❖ **Creating a positive work environment:** Creating a positive work atmosphere improves self-confidence and results in strong professional connections. This can contribute to the development of respect, professionalism, and confidence.

III. Communication and Relationship with Team Members

Health care delivery is a team effort and is the process of achieving a goal through collaboration with a group of individuals. Each team member performs a crucial function and is interdependent on the other team members for various elements of patient care. Some team members aid in disease diagnosis, while others specialize in specific elements of patient care, such as physical and emotional requirements. While working as a team member, communication skills are vital for nurses, but they can be tough to master. The level of communication between nurses and other members of the team has a significant impact on health outcomes. Therefore, a nurse must always strive to enhance his or her communication abilities, as poor communication can be harmful and lead to problems.

Strategies to improve communication among team members
- ❖ Active listening without interrupting the conveyed facts.
- ❖ Conveying an accepting attitude and empathy.
- ❖ Showing genuine interest by staying focused on the conversation.
- ❖ Use non-verbal body language of interest and concern such as leaning forward, listening carefully, maintaining eye contact, etc.
- ❖ Offering factual information and avoiding conveying of false assurance.
- ❖ Using reflection and restating the feelings and spoken words.

Strategies to improve the positive relationship with team members
- ❖ *Open communication:* Open communication always improves the relationship among the members as it avoids conflicts. Members must be able to effectively communicate with each other to overcome obstacles, and resolve conflict.
- ❖ *Effective coordination:* Effective coordination results in efficient cooperation among the members of the health care team. This avoids confusion and helps in achieving desired outcomes as it maintains high levels of trust among the members.
- ❖ *Commitment and cohesiveness:* The equal distribution of work and working as a cohesive team for the welfare of the patients promotes a sense of commitment and cohesion among the members of the team.

Respectful and Open Communication

Respectful communication is crucial for a healthy workplace atmosphere. Creating a culture that encourages good, effective, and courteous communication in the nursing profession can promote teamwork, efficiency, and cohesion. Open communication is readily sharing information between people in a transparent, honest, consistent, and dependable way. When team members openly communicate, they express their thoughts, feelings, emotions, and plans clearly and assertively. Open communication happens in a team when its members are empowered to share their thoughts without any fear of rejection or disapproval.

The following are the challenges of professionalism in nursing that can arise while encountering professional relationships with team members of the health care system:

- **Use of inclusive language:** The use of inappropriate language that may discriminate against a person based on color, caste, religion, gender identity, etc., is always a threat to professionalism. Further, aggressive, passive, or passive-aggressive words also hamper professional interactions. Consequently, it is the primary obligation of each member to provide respect, decency, and thoughtfulness in personal and professional relationships.
- **Body language and non-verbal cues:** Nonverbal cues including eye contact, smiling, facial expressions, attitude, etc., play a significant part in the effective transmission of information among team members. Movements, such as fidgeting express disinterest and hinder the professional relationship.
- **Being dishonest and untruthful:** The foundation of a respectful professional relationship is honesty and impartiality. Adopting a disrespectful attitude will break down team cohesion and trust among the team members. The nurse should guarantee that they are stating the truth when delivering information.
- **Problems in communication dialogues:** Too much criticism often results in undesirable conduct or activity. However, requesting the team members to engage in different activities fosters positivity and respect.

Strategies for achieving respectful and open communication in nursing

- **R**–recognize the work or efforts of other members
- **E**–encourage open communication and listen to others
- **S**–speak directly with the person rather than talking about them to others
- **P**–practice kindness and politeness
- **E**–empathy and emotionality for others
- **C**–consider dissenting opinions or disagreements of others
- **T**–treat everyone fairly and equally

IV. Communication and Relationship with Team Members about Relevant Interests for Ethical Decision-making

Ethics are the principles that guide a person's behavior which will differ from person to person. While making ethical decisions, the nurse has to consider both the personal beliefs and moral standards of the other members of the team. Ethical decision-making is the process of evaluating and selecting alternatives following ethical ideals. To make ethical decisions, it is required to recognize and eliminate immoral alternatives and choose the most ethical option.

Throughout nursing careers, ethical dilemmas are arising in a variety of scenarios. This can be quite stressful as we strive to determine the correctness of action in the context of a specific situation. The following are the challenges for the nurses when encountering certain ethical decision-making situations while working as a team member in the health care system:

- **Respect for human dignity:** Respecting human dignity is sometimes a challenge for the nurses while rendering service. For example, the ethical dilemma while assisting a client in the abortion is a challenge for the nurse depending on their cultural and religious background.
- **Non-maleficence:** The duty of non-maleficence places the members of the profession not to be an agent of harm. The ethical principle of 'do no harm' operates at several levels depending upon the various contexts. For example, assisting a case of physician-assisted dying or euthanasia is a great matter of ethical dilemma among nurses while upholding the principle of 'do no harm'.
- **Beneficence:** The principle of beneficence highlights that all the members of the health care team have a moral obligation to provide optimum care to all kinds of patients.
- **Truth-telling:** Many health professionals have the opinion that patients need professionals who always help them to maintain hope in their distress. However, it is worth noting that truth-telling, is often an ethical dilemma for nurses while conveying bad news to patients and families.
- **Autonomy:** This enables nurses to appreciate and support a patient's decision to accept or reject life-sustaining treatments. Nurses' role as patient advocates is to ensure that patients are adequately informed about the potential risks, benefits, and

complications of their treatment. Many elements, such as culture, age, client's present mental health status, and the social support system, might impact the patient's acceptance or refusal of medical treatment.
- **Informed consent:** Sometimes, obtaining informed consent can be a difficult ethical dilemma. For example, after informing about the potential risk of any procedure, a patient might be in a dilemma of whether to accept or reject the treatment.
- **Protecting patient privacy and confidentiality:** Privacy and confidentiality of patients are important ethical concerns for nurses. This might have legal implications and result in serious penalties for healthcare personnel if not performed correctly.
- **Inadequate resources and staffing:** Although this is not an ethical issue that can be blamed on individual nurses, a shortage of resources and inadequate personnel in the area of patient care forces nurses to make difficult judgements in some cases. If there is not enough staff to care for all of the patients, patient care will be compromised.

Dealing with Ethical Issues in Nursing

Dealing with ethical dilemmas is a difficult task for nurses. Nurses are frequently confronted with several questions about medical treatments and may fail or succeed in responding to these ethical challenges. The work experience and interaction with other members of the team, patients, and their relatives can help nurses understand how to respond to these problems. They should speak honestly about the best decision for the patient while remaining open to disagreements. Reviewing the professional code of ethics and determining a solution to one's specific situation is the best response to ethical difficulties in nursing. Respectful and open communication is the only way to overcome the challenges of ethical decision-making.

V. Relationship with Patients and Society

The patients are the most crucial member of the health team; without them, there would be no team at all. Rapid changes are taking place in methods and procedures in nursing due to scientific developments. However, the main objective of nursing care remains the same which includes the provision of quality care centered upon the health needs of the patient and family. The nurses who are committed to uphold the profession face certain barriers while striving to work for professionalism within the relationships that they encounter. The following are the three challenges of professionalism in nursing that can arise while encountering professional relationships with patients and society:

- ❖ **Conduct-related issues:** A professional relationship is always the product of right conduct between the patient and the health care provider. Conduct refers to the acceptable standards of behavior, actions, beliefs, and moral practices. Professional conduct refers to the set of expected behaviors while acting in the professional areas of nursing. However, different aspects, such as age, gender, employment, social background, and moral and religious values between the nurse and the patient determine the patterns of appropriate and inappropriate behavior. Because of these discrepancies, the nurse is unable to fully comprehend the patient's behaviors and reactions.
- ❖ **Attitude and inherent traits related issues:** A positive attitude and praiseworthy character traits results in an enduring professional relationship with the patient. The strength of nurse-client relationship is influenced by the judgement about the personality traits and attitudes they possess. For example, expectations of society towards the nursing profession would be respect and dignity while meeting their health care needs. However, this largely depends on the individual traits of the professionals involved in it.
- ❖ **Context-related issues:** The individual, social, and institutional context is an influencing factor that determines the professional relationship. The emotional or physical condition of patients and family members may make it difficult for them to understand the totality of the imposed limitations within the treatment process which might hamper the nurse-client relationship. For example, a heavy workload and shortage of manpower create disturbances in the nurse-client relationship.

Measures to Demonstrate a Professional Relationship with Patients and Society

In a professional relationship, the nurse must ascertain certain qualities to build a successful interaction with the patients and society.
- ❖ **Simplicity:** Concise use of communication without using difficult or unfamiliar terms always promotes professional relationship.

- ❖ **Clarity:** Clarity in actions and reactions is very important for supporting a professional relationship.
- ❖ **Relevance:** Acting upon the relevant needs of the patient within the professional boundaries fosters a healthy relationship.
- ❖ **Adaptability:** The nurse has to consider the whole aspects of the unmet healthcare needs of the client and adapt the response that favors the patient.
- ❖ **Respect:** Validation and accurate interpretation of the actual and potential health problems eliminate misunderstanding and develop mutual respect and dignity.

CHAPTER HIGHLIGHTS

- ❖ Profession and occupation are different in more general sense.
- ❖ A profession possesses certain characteristics and criteria.
- ❖ Nursing is a profession as it has all the characteristics of a profession and fulfills all its criteria.
- ❖ Nurses have expanded educational and career roles in addition to their patient care roles.
- ❖ Professionalism means the act of behaving in a manner that is expected by a profession.
- ❖ Maintaining personal identity and professional identity, self-integrity, communication and relationship with team members especially in times of ethical dilemmas, the patients and the society are major challenges of professionalism in nursing.
- ❖ Nurses should adapt certain strategies like creating a professional image, being honest and accountable, listening actively, having respectful and open communication, protecting patient privacy, confidentiality etc., to promote professionalism.

MULTIPLE CHOICE QUESTIONS

1. What is the meaning of the word 'profession'?
    - a. 'to proclaim something publicly'
    - b. 'to lead out'
    - c. 'to move out'
    - d. 'to procaste'
2. The following are the characteristics of a profession as compared to occupation, *except:*
    - a. Code of conduct is essential
    - b. A regulated body is present
    - c. Formal training is not mandatory
    - d. Values and beliefs are essential

3. Which of the following are the criteria for a profession?
   a. Body of knowledge
   b. Altruism
   c. Formal education
   d. All of the above
4. The meaning of the word 'nursing' includes:
   a. 'to help'
   b. 'to nurture'
   c. 'to support'
   d. 'provide care'
5. Which of the following is a challenge to professionalism?
   a. Preservation of self-integrity
   b. Communication and relationship with team members
   c. Relationship with patients and society
   d. All of the above

ANSWERS

1. a   2. c   3. d   4. b   5. d

BIBLIOGRAPHY

1. Alidina K. Professionalism in post-licensure nurses in developed countries. Journal of Nursing Education and Practice. 2013 May 1;3(5):128.
2. Berman A, Snyder SJ, Levett-Jones T, Dwyer T, Hales M, Harvey N, Moxham L, Langtree T, Parker B, Reid-Searl K, Stanley D. Kozier and Erb's Fundamentals of Nursing [4th Australian edition].
3. Black B. Professional nursing e-book: Concepts & challenges. Elsevier Health Sciences. 2019 Jun 26.
4. Burton MA, Ludwig LJ. Fundamentals of nursing care: concepts, connections & skills. FA Davis. 2014 Oct 10.
5. Chitty KK, Black BP. Professional nursing: concepts & challenges. 3rd ed. Philadelphia: Saunders. 2001.
6. Cruess RL, Cruess SR, Johnston SE. Professionalism: an ideal to be sustained. Lancet. 2000 Jul 8;356(9224):156-9.
7. Fitzgerald A. Professional identity: A concept analysis. Nursing Forum. 2020; 55 (3); 447-472.
8. Ghadirian F, Salsali M, Cheraghi MA. Nursing professionalism: An evolutionary concept analysis. Iranian Journal of Nursing and Midwifery Research. 2014; 19(1): 1-10.
9. Hoeve Y, Jansen G, Roodbol P. The nursing profession: public image, self-concept, and professional identity. A discussion paper. J Adv Nurs. 2014 Feb;70(2):295-309. Available from https://pubmed.ncbi.nlm.nih.gov/23711235/. doi: 10.1111/jan.12177.
10. Kanniyakonil S. The Fundamentals of Bioethics: Legal Perspectives and Ethical Aproches. Scaria Kanniyakonil. 2007.

11. Liebles JG, Mc Commel RC. Management Principles for Health Professionals, Fourth edition, Massachusetts: Jones and Bartlett Publishers. 2004.
12. Potter PA, Perry AG, Hall AE, Stockert PA. Fundamentals of nursing. Elsevier mosby. 2009.
13. Pullen, Richard L. Professional identity in nursing practice. Nursing Made Incredibly Easy! 2021 Apr 19(2):55-56.
14. Shohani M, Zamanzadeh V. Nurses' Attitude towards Professionalization and Factors Influencing it. Journal of Caring Science. 2017; 6(4) 345–357.
15. Sibiya MN. Effective communication in nursing. Nursing. 2018 Mar 21;19:20-34.
16. Vati J. Principles and Practice of Nursing Management and Administration: For BSc and MSc Nursing (as Per the Syllabus of Indian Nursing Council). Jaypee Brothers Medical Publishers. 2013.
17. Vivekananda-Schmidt P, Crossley J, Murdoch-Eaton D. A model of professional self-identity formation in student doctors and dentists: a mixed method study. BMC Med Educ. 2015; 15:83.
18. Warnock LG. Reflecting principles of Professionalism. Canadian Journal of Surgery. 2008; 51(2): 84–85.

CHAPTER 2

Professional Conduct

Biji P Varkey, Deepak

Learning Objectives

Upon completion of this chapter, the student should be able to:
- Discuss meaning, purposes, and code of professional conduct
- Describe ethical principles and professional conduct
- Illustrate importance of adherence to policies, rules, and regulations of the institutions
- Elaborate professional etiquettes and behaviors
- Highlight importance of professional grooming

■ PROFESSIONAL CONDUCT

Conduct refers to the acceptable standards of behavior, actions, beliefs, and moral practices. Professional conduct refers to the set of expected behaviours while acting in the professional areas of nursing. The code of professional conduct is a series of statements for guiding professional accountability, competency, and the quality of professional practice. These are the legal documents that provide a framework for professionally accountable behaviors. Therefore, a breach of professional conduct is considered a matter of professional misconduct. Professional conduct represents the minimum requirements of the profession, such as the range of roles, functions, and related professional activities. The code of professional conduct helps in enhancing high-quality services while performing responsibilities in various areas, such as clinical practice including nursing administration, education, and research. They serve as a reference guide regarding the ethical obligations that are expected from the nurses while rendering their services within the nursing profession.

Purposes of Code of Professional Conduct

The following are the purposes of the code of professional conduct:
- To promote safe and effective practice among nurses.
- To create an expected standard of conduct for the nursing profession.
- To inform the public about the minimum standards for the professional conduct of nurses.
- To generate a reliable document for decisions involving ethical guidelines for professional behavior.
- To empower the nursing personnel to be accountable for their well-being and actions.
- To identify the minimum obligations in practice and professional relationships.

Code of Professional Conduct for Nurses in India

In India, there are six codes of professional conduct for nurses. Each code is accompanied by certain subsidiary statements regarding the standards of conduct providing further information about the code **(Refer Table 2.1 and Fig. 2.1).**

TABLE 2.1: Code of professional conduct.

1. Professional responsibility and accountability	Explanation
As members of the professions, nurse must	
1.1 Appreciates and nurtures one's sense of worth	A sense of *self-respect* is a fundamental value to uphold personal and professional integrity
1.2 Upholds moral standards that are commendable to the profession	The nurse must maintain *personal behaviors, attitudes, and actions* within the scope of practice
1.3 Fulfills obligations within the parameters of one's professional boundaries	The nurse must be responsible and accountable for all the decisions and actions in one's professional practice
1.4 Is responsible for upholding the Indian Nursing Council's practice standards	
1.5 Is responsible for one's actions and decisions	

Contd...

Unit 1: Professionals in Nursing

Contd...

1.6 Is sympathetic	The nurse must enhance the interest of patients by helping them according to their requirements
1.7 Responsible for ensuring that current practices are continually improved	The nurse must update one's professional knowledge and skills to ensure evidence-based practice.
1.8 Gives people enough information so they can make informed decisions	The nurse must communicate the possible options and anticipate treatments according to the level of understanding of the client and relatives
1.9 Demonstrates healthy habits	The nurse must work for safeguarding and protect patients' rights and individual rights and maintains professional relationship at all levels
2. Nursing practice	**Explanation**
As members of the professions, nurses must	
2.1 Conforms to established standards of practice in providing care	The nurse must ensure the essential quality of care while rendering service without compromising the client's safety
2.2 Provides care in the areas of physical, psychological, emotional, social, and spiritual care while treating all people and families with respect for human dignity	The nurse must ensure the provision of culturally congruent care with human dignity intending to promote healthy practices in the patients and their families
2.3 Respects people and their families from the perspective of customs and culture, fostering healthy habits and avoiding harmful ones	
2.4 Helps people and families make autonomous decisions by presenting a factually accurate and complete picture in all circumstances	The nurse must truthfully discuss the treatment plans and helps to provide the choices for accepting or refusing the treatment decisions
2.5 Encourages individuals and close family members to participate in the care of others in the care	
2.6 Assures safe conduct	The nurse must practice in a *'safe and competent manner'* to protect themself and their patients
2.7 When a patient's care needs exceed what the nurse is capable of handling, she consults, coordinates collaborate and follow up as necessary	The nurse must seek professional advice, or guidance from their superior or concerned authorities wherever required

Contd...

Contd...

3. Communication and interpersonal relationships	Explanation
As members of the professions, nurses must	
3.1 Develops and upholds successful relationships with people, families, and societies	The nurse must practice reflectively and maintain appropriate communications and therapeutic relationships with patients and their family members
3.2 Respects the worth of teammates and uphold healthy interpersonal relationships with them	
3.3 Respects and encourages team members' contributions to profession	The nurse must ensure the delivery of healthcare services in coordination with the multidisciplinary team to meet the health needs of the clients and families
3.4 Meets the needs of individuals, families, and communities in collaboration with other healthcare professionals	

4. Valuing human being	Explanation
As members of the professions, nurses must	
4.1 Takes the necessary steps to safeguard people from unethical conduct that is harmful	The nurse must act lawfully and initiate supporting actions in the best interest of individuals
4.2 Thinks about pertinent information while making moral decisions that are in people's best interests.	
4.3 Encourages individuals to exercise their right to speak out on matters affecting their well-being	The nurse must advocate for patient safety and well-being in all circumstances
4.4 Respects and encourages personal decision-making	

5. Management	Explanation
As members of the professions, nurses must	
5.1 Makes sure that resources are used and allocated properly	The nurse must be efficient to make the best use of available resources to maintain cost-effective care
5.2 Supervises and teaches students and other formal healthcare workers while doing so	The nurse is responsible to educate students and other care providers on the values, principles, and standards of health care

Contd...

Contd...

5.3 Makes decisions based on individual competency while having to accept and assign responsibility	Nurse has the responsibility to support and guide the team members to promote the "we feeling" without compromising the quality of care
5.4 Helps to create a conducive work environment to accomplish institutional goals	
5.5 Utilizes suitable channels of communication to effectively communicate	
5.6 Takes part in the appraisal system	The nurse must ensure consistency in the continuous evaluation of nursing services to meet the quality of care
5.7 Takes part in the assessment of nursing services	
5.8 Takes part in policy-making while adhering to the principle of service equity and accessibility	The nurse must be involved in policy decisions and assertive about the proper allocation of funds to uphold the quality of the profession
5.9 Works with people to determine their needs and educates funding and policy-making organizations about resource allocation	
6. Professional advancement	**Explanation**
As members of the professions, nurses must	
6.1 Maintains respect for human rights while working to further the improvement of knowledge	The nurse must ensure that professional advancement is matched with the patient's preferences and values
6.2 Supports the advancement of nursing practice	The nurse must engage in activities that build a framework for nursing practice
6.3 Participates in deciding and putting into practice quality care	The nurse must engage in professional advancement through continuous learning, implementing quality control services, and participating in evidence-based research
6.4 Assumes responsibility for keeping knowledge and skills up to date	
6.5 Conducts and participates in research to advance the fundamental knowledge of their field	

■ ETHICAL PRINCIPLES AND PROFESSIONAL CONDUCT

Ethics is a broad term that covers the study of the moral principles that govern a person to decide the rightness and wrongness of an action. It is a branch of philosophy that deals with moral principles or moral values. Therefore, it is also called moral philosophy.

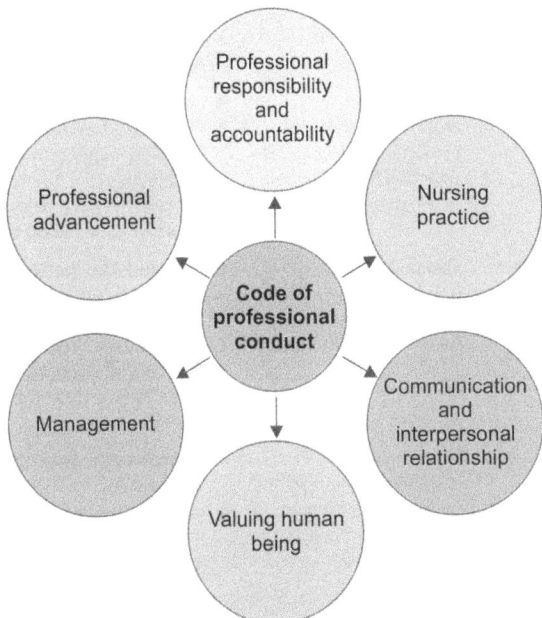

Fig. 2.1: Code of professional conduct for nurses in India.

The inhumane experimentation in World War II leads to the evolution of bioethics as a part of professional conduct in the health care sciences with extensive scopes in the areas, such as research ethics, clinical ethics, etc. There are four fundamental principles of ethics: Beneficence, nonmaleficence, autonomy, and justice **(Refer Fig. 2.2 and Table 2.2).**

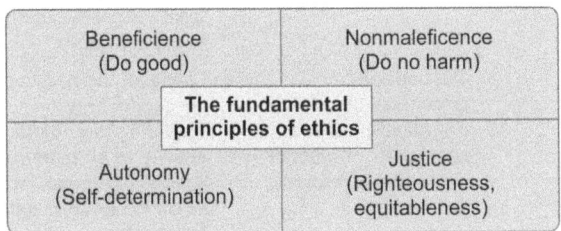

Fig. 2.2: Fundamental principles of ethics.

TABLE 2.2: Ethical principles.

Ethical principles	Meaning	Areas of professional conduct
Beneficence	This principle emphasizes the importance of '*do good*' or acting for the benefit of the patient	❖ Defend the rights of the patient ❖ To help the person when he needed especially those with disabilities ❖ To help the persons experiencing harm or anticipating danger
Nonmaleficence	This principle emphasizes the importance of 'do no harm' or prevent harm	❖ Helping the patient to select the best course of action and avoiding inappropriate burdens ❖ Avoiding the unintended harmful effects of drugs or certain difficult situations such as the end of life care decisions.
Autonomy	This principle emphasizes the right to determine for own treatment or choices of actions (self-determination)	❖ Accepting the patients' rights and preferences ❖ Informed consent: Disclosing the information of the treatment or procedure before conducting a medical or surgical procedure or research. The requirements for informed consent are (a) the patient received a full disclosure or knowledge about the procedure, (b) the patient is competent enough for the procedure, and (c) the patient acts voluntarily to consent to the procedure ❖ Truth-telling: This is the act of communicating the facts without falseness or deceit. This will improve the *trust* between the nurse and the patient ❖ Confidentiality: This is the act of keeping the information given by the client within the health care team and not disclosing the same to any third party
Justice	This principle emphasizes the fairness or equitableness and appropriate distribution of health care resources and services.	❖ Caring for the patient as per the needs or priority ❖ Providing standards of care equally to all patients without considering certain factors, such as socioeconomic status, caste, religion, etc.

■ **Critical Thinking**
What are the situations in which there is a breach of confidentiality that is not considered a violation of ethical principles in the health care setting?

ADHERENCE TO POLICIES, RULES, AND REGULATIONS OF THE INSTITUTIONS

Following policies and standards of the statutory bodies, rules and regulations of the institutions, and protocols of the units/departments are the indicators of professional conduct. The nurse must understand their role and responsibilities concerning their professional conduct set by the concerned statutory body. The nursing profession is pressured to adapt to external expectations from the changing society and therefore, the content of professional conduct needs to be frequently evaluated. Ensuring the practice of professional standards helps the nurse to be adherent to the regulations and it further promotes human dignity. Certain factors need to be considered while understanding professional conduct and policies and regulations of the institutions. These include internal factors, such as individual personalities, responsibilities, and communication obstacles, as well as external factors, such as institutional prerequisites and support systems.

Internal Factors

- **Individual character and responsibility:** The individual character is unique to that individual that includes the sum of behaviors and acts of thinking in their daily life situations. The character is relatively formed during childhood and the surrounding environment has a vital influence in changing the same. A nurse has to encounter various unpredictable challenges in her professional practice which need possession of positive energy to tackle the situations. With encouragement and empowerment, one can expect a proper adherence to professional conduct.
- **Communication challenges:** Adherence to professional conduct is mediated by some communication challenges, such as communication between nurses and other health care professionals, the professional relationship among employees, nurse-patient relationship. The acquisition of certain internal

skills, such as communicating assertively can help in providing efficient care without compromising professional conduct.

External Factors

- **Institutional pre-conditions:** The equipment and facilities used in hospitals are crucial in ensuring that professional conduct is followed. Inappropriate nurse-patient ratio, heavy workload, and deploying the work area without considering the experience of the nurse are the common indicators of non-adherence to professional conduct.
- **Support systems:** A sound system of rewards and penalties could improve the experience of professional behavior. Flexibility in the working conditions and appropriate support systems are important factors of proper adherence to rules and regulations.

PROFESSIONAL ETIQUETTES AND BEHAVIORS

Etiquette is the various manners and behaviors prescribed by a particular society. Professional etiquettes are the polite behaviors acceptable among the members of a profession. Every person has his or her own unique set of manners and behaviors that includes both acceptable and unprofessional aspects. The following are the several aspects of professional etiquette and behaviors that are important to the nursing profession:

- **Posture:** Posture reflects the confidence level attitude, as well as the interest, and has important implications in establishing therapeutic relationships. Maintaining the SOLER technique is a good therapeutic tool during the nurse-client relationship for ensuring active listening.
    - S - Sitting in a comfortable position facing the client. This posture conveys the message that the nurse is ready to listen.
    - O - Ensure an *open posture* by avoiding crossing arms or legs.
    - L - Leaning toward the client indicates the message of eagerness and genuine interest in the interaction.
    - E - Establishing eye contact encourages the client to continue the therapeutic interaction.
    - R - Remaining relaxed promotes the comfort of the client.

❖ **Mastery in the use of language:** The mastery of delivering grammatically proper, professional, and polite language is one of the most important etiquettes required in the professional setting. Table 2.3 presents commonly used unprofessional language and their better professional alternatives.

TABLE 2.3: Use of unprofessional language and the relevant professional alternative.

Language: Unprofessional use	Professional alternative
What's up?	How are you?
What do you want?	How may I help you?
I don't understand what you said	Please clarify what you mean.
What?	Pardon? Excuse me?

❖ **Avoiding distracting behaviors:** Some distracting behaviors may hinder professionalism and must be avoided. The unacceptable etiquettes while in the professional setting are depicted in Table 2.4.

TABLE 2.4: Distracting behaviors and possible solutions.

Distracting behaviors in the professional setting	Possible solutions
Using chewing gums	Bad breath can be avoided by ensuring proper dental care and not by chewing gum
Using snack items	Snack items should be consumed out of the sight of the patient
Using cigarettes/alcohol	Ensure that the patients and health team members should never smell cigarette smoke/alcohol breath as it is highly offensive
Using electronic gadgets	All portable devices such as mobile phones should be turned off or silenced while in the professional setting
Use of social media	A professional must always create a positive image of oneself while using social media. This can be maintained by avoiding inappropriate profile images, avoiding bad language or written content, etc.

■ PROFESSIONAL GROOMING: UNIFORM, DRESS CODE

All healthcare personnel is required to keep up adequate standards of personal grooming and to always present a clean, professional appearance. The nursing staff's uniform and dress code can affect the clients' level of safety as well as how the general public views their professionalism and the caliber of their services. Therefore, nurses who interact with patients, their families, or the general public are required to dress professionally.

Purposes

- To contribute to the safety of both clients and nurses as it helps in avoiding the malpractice.
- To raise public expectations as well as the regard, believe, and confidence of the patient.
- To support infection prevention and control practices.
- To adhere to standards of professional appearance.

General Guidelines

- The uniform or the dress code must be clean and maintained hygienically to represent a professional appearance appropriate to the nursing profession.
- All inappropriate clothing should be avoided, such as stained, soiled, too tight-fitting dresses, revealing dresses, etc.,
- Depending on the area of involvement, adherence to a certain uniform is mandatory. For example, an ICU nurse would wear clothing up to the elbow for facilitating regular hand hygiene practices.
- Gowns or other barrier-protective clothing may not be worn for any other reason or outside of a professional context. However, it can be acceptable while attending a clinical emergency.
- Footwear must be clean and safe as per the areas of posting.
- Jewelry, buttons, pins, and other accessories and ornaments must be limited.
- The cosmetics should be appropriate to the professional setting and avoid the use of perfumes with noticeable scents.
- Hair should be clean, neatly styled, and must adhere to occupational standards and infection control policies.
- While on duty, nurses are required to wear and make visible photo identification badges or other forms of identification.
- Maintaining cleanliness and good personal hygiene are crucial for projecting a favorable and professional image to clients and their families.

■ **Critical Thinking**
Does professional grooming help in delivering better patient care?

■ PROFESSIONAL BOUNDARIES: PROFESSIONAL RELATIONSHIP WITH THE PATIENTS, CAREGIVERS, AND TEAM MEMBERS

Professional boundaries are the socially constructed limits that establish the therapeutic relationship among patients, caregivers, nurses, and other health care team members. It provides a framework for what is, and what is not expected in a professional relationship. Professional boundaries form the secure foundation for nursing personnel to build and maintain therapeutic relationships with clients and their caregivers. Working within professional boundaries helps to promote trust among the patients and health care team. Professional boundaries help in fostering the key elements of the nurse-patient relationship, such as trust, mutual respect, and empathy.

Professional Boundary Violation

Boundary violations are the activities that deviate from an established boundary while engaging in a professional relationship. The following are the activities of boundary violation in the therapeutic relationship (**Fig. 2.3**):

* **Sharing personal information:** Discussing intimate personal problems and issues with the patient may end up in personal relationships than professional relationships.
* **Non-therapeutic touch:** Non-therapeutic touch is part of boundary violation as it will not serve any good purpose or meet the needs of the client.
* **Giving or accepting gifts:** Giving or receiving gifts is not acceptable in the therapeutic relationship as it leads to more personal than professionals.

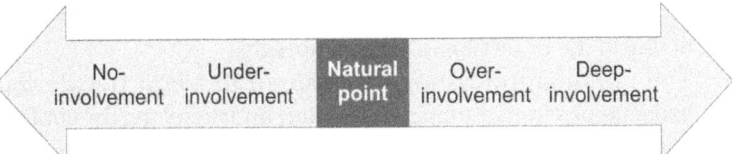

Fig. 2.3: Continuum of professional relationship.

- **Over-involvement or under-involvement:** To maintain professional boundaries, the nurse should neither over-involved nor under-involved while encountering professional relationships. Examples of over-involvement include spending too much time with one particular client, visiting clients at inappropriate times, and showing favoritism. Under-involvement may be manifested in the form of neglect, dishonesty, etc.
- **Romantic relationships and sexual misconduct:** Remaining in a romantic or sexual relationship with the patient is an extreme violation of professional boundaries charged with the legal offense.

Strategies to Overcome or Prevent Boundary Violation in the Professional Relationship

The nurses have an important role to work within the professional boundaries while fulfilling the physical care and emotional needs of the client. The following are some of the strategies to maintain professional boundaries in the therapeutic relationship:

- Clarify the professional roles and objectives of the therapeutic relationship at the beginning of therapeutic interaction as applicable.
- Set verbal boundaries by using therapeutic communication techniques.
- Set appropriate physical boundaries such as maintaining a therapeutic physical distance while ensuring care, maintaining professional etiquette, and polite behavior.
- Document the interactions and discussions with subordinates and supervisors in case they experience any unfavorable situations.
- Maintain respect and privacy in every therapeutic interaction.
- Be aware and understand the consequences of boundary violations.

■ CHAPTER HIGHLIGHTS

- Professional conduct refers to the set of expected behaviors while acting in the professional areas of nursing.
- The nursing profession is pressured to adapt to external expectations from the changing society and therefore, the content of professional conduct needs to be frequently evaluated.
- Professional etiquettes are the polite behaviors acceptable among the members of a profession.

- All healthcare personnel is required to keep up adequate standards of personal grooming and to always present a clean, professional appearance.
- Professional boundaries are the socially constructed limits that establish the therapeutic relationship among patients, caregivers, nurses, and other health care team members.

MULTIPLE CHOICE QUESTIONS

1. The series of statements for guiding the professional accountability, competency, and the quality of professional practice are:
   a. Professional etiquettes
   b. Professional conduct
   c. Professional ethics
   d. Professional boundaries
2. Which of the following is NOT included in the code of professional conduct for nurses in India?
   a. Professional accountability
   b. Professional advancement
   c. Nursing education
   d. Nursing management
3. Which of the following is NOT considered fundamental principles of ethics?
   a. Beneficence
   b. Autonomy
   c. Justice
   d. Veracity
4. The polite behaviors acceptable among the members of a profession are called as:
   a. Professional etiquettes
   b. Professional conduct
   c. Professional ethics
   d. Professional boundaries
5. Which of the following is considered a matter of boundary violation in the therapeutic relationship?
   a. Over-involvement
   b. Accepting gifts
   c. Non-therapeutic touch
   d. All of the above

ANSWERS

1. b   2. c   3. d   4. a   5. d

BIBLIOGRAPHY

1. Aylott M. Blurring the boundaries: Technology and the nurse-patient relationship. British Journal of Nursing. 2011 Jul 12;20(13):810-6.
2. Beauchamp C. Beauchamp TL, Childress JF. Principles of biomedical ethics. New York (NY): Oxford University Press. 2009; pp. 162–4.
3. Bladh ML, Van Leeuwen AM. Nurse-to-patient etiquette: It's more than good manners. Nursing2020. 2017 Aug 1;47(8):52-6.

4. Code of ethics and professional Conduct: Indian Nursing Council Available from: https://vspmmdine.edu.in/wp-content/uploads/2022/04/7.1.9-web-link-of-code-of-conduct.pdf [Last accessed on 02/05/2022]
5. Day LJ. Nursing care of potential organ donors: An articulation of ethics, etiquette and practice. University of California, San Francisco. 1999.
6. Hall K. Professional boundaries: Building a trusting relationship with patients. Home Healthcare Now. 2011 Apr 1;29(4):210-7.
7. Johnstone MJ. Bioethics: A nursing perspective. Elsevier Health Sciences. 2019 May 31.
8. Jonsen AR, Siegler M, Winslade WJ. Clinical ethics a practical approach to ethical decisions in clinical medicine. McGraw Hill. 2015, 8th edition.
9. Kangasniemi M, Pakkanen P, Korhonen A. Professional ethics in nursing: An integrative review. Journal of advanced nursing. 2015 Aug;71(8):1744-57.
10. National Council of State Boards of Nursing. A Nurse's Guide to Professional Boundaries. Chicago, IL: NCSBN; 2011. Available from: https://www.ncsbn.org/ProfessionalBoundaries_Complete.pdf [Last accessed on 02/05/2022]
11. Pagana KD. Etiquette & Communication Strategies for Nurses. Sigma. 2019 Nov 8.
12. Perry CM. Nursing ethics and etiquette. The American Journal of Nursing. 1906 Apr 1;6(7):448-52.
13. Peternelj-Taylor CA, Yonge O. Exploring boundaries in the nurse-client relationship: Professional roles and responsibilities. Perspectives in Psychiatric Care. 2003 Apr;39(2):55-66.
14. Safdar SA, Aqeel L. Grooming and etiquette as part of nurse's professionalism: An essential curricular competency. Pakistan Journal of Medical Sciences. 2019 Mar;35(2):404.
15. Slobogian V, Giles J, Rent T. Boundaries: When patients become friends. Canadian Oncology Nursing Journal. 2017;27(4).394.
16. Thompson HO, Thompson JE. Code of ethics for nurse-midwives. Journal of Nurse-Midwifery. 1986 Mar 1;31(2):99-102.
17. Varkey B. Principles of clinical ethics and their application to practice. Medical Principles and Practice. 2021;30(1):17-28.
18. Vijayalakshmi P, Narayanan A, Thankachan A, Changhorla, A, SaiNikhil Reddy S. Professional and ethical values in Nursing practice: An Indian Perspective. Invest. Educ. Enferm. 2021; 39(2):e12.
19. Wills NL, Wilson B, Woodcock EB, Abraham SP, Gillum DR. Appearance of nurses and perceived professionalism. International Journal of Studies in Nursing. 2018 Jul 30;3(3):30.

CHAPTER 3

Regulatory Bodies and Professional Organization

Urvashi Goyal, Jaison Joseph

Learning Objectives

Upon completion of this chapter, the student should be able to:
- Understand the regulatory bodies of the nursing profession in India.
- Discuss different national and international professional nursing organizations.
- Describe activities and functioning of regulatory bodies and professional organizations.

REGULATORY BODIES: ROLES AND RESPONSIBILITIES

A regulatory body is a formal institution, established by statute or by an authorized government agency that implements the regulatory process as a means of bringing order, uniformity, and control to a profession and its practice. **Figure 3.1** represents the purposes of professional bodies in nursing.

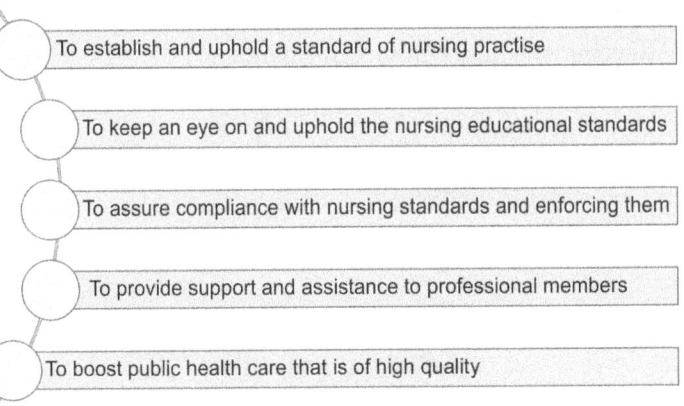

Fig. 3.1: Purposes of the regulatory bodies in nursing.

Indian Nursing Council

The Indian Nursing Council was created by the Government of India under section 3(1) of the Indian Nursing Council Act, 1947, of parliament to create a uniform standard of training for nurses, midwives, and health visitors. It is an independent body that reports to the Ministry of Health and Family Welfare of the Government of India. **Figure 3.2** represents the organizational hierarchy of the Indian Nursing Council.

Functions of the Indian Nursing Council

- Develop and sustain a uniform standard of nursing education for nurses, midwives, ANMs, and health visitors through inspections of nursing programs.
- To acknowledge the requirements outlined in Section 10(2)(4) of the Indian Nursing Council Act, 1947, for registration and employment both within India and abroad.
- Permission to register nurses with foreign degrees who are Indian or foreign citizens under section 11(2)(a) of the Indian Nursing Council Act, 1947.
- To specify minimum requirements for education and training in programs offered as well as to specify nursing program curricula and rules.
- The power to withdraw recognition of training institute if standards are not maintained.
- To guide a variety of issues relating to nursing education in the nation to the State Nursing Councils, Examining Boards, State Governments, and Central Government.

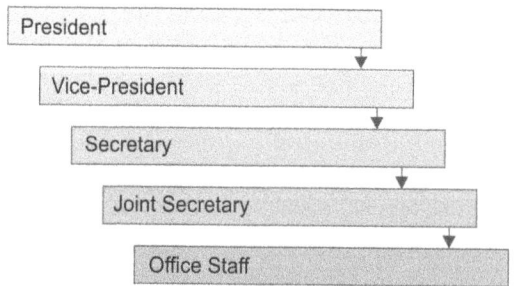

Fig. 3.2: Organizational structure of Indian Nursing Council.

- Recognize organizations, and institutions that offer Masters, Bachelors, Postgraduate Diplomas, Diplomas, and Certificate Programs in Nursing for suitability as per standards.
- To advance nursing research.
- To maintain a registry of Indian nurses for the registration of nursing personnel.
- Regular revision of curriculum for the nursing courses.
- Plan and approval of new nursing education programs for execution as per the need of the country.

State Nursing Council

The State Nursing Council, an independent organization with official recognition, has the authority to enact state laws governing both licensed nurses and nurses enrolled in various educational programmes. Despite operating independently, the state nursing council needs the state government's permission before passing any laws or making any decisions about the nursing profession.

Functions of State Nursing Council

- To inspect and accredit nursing schools in their state.
- Assessment and evaluation of various nursing programmes
- Establish codes of conduct and implement punishments for violations.
- Keeping a register of nurses, midwives, and health visitors.
- Registration of nurses and midwives in their states.

■ **Critical Thinking**
1. What can be done to promote professional conduct among nursing professionals?

■ PROFESSIONAL ORGANIZATION

A professional organization is also referred to as a professional body or association that aids in the advancement of a profession, promotes the general welfare, and safeguards the interests of its members who work in that profession. It encourages teamwork, connections among members of the organization, and invention. It has an elected leadership body, as well as several subcommittees or working divisions. Professional associations can be regional, national, or international in scope, and they typically have relations to universities and institutions that offer relevant degree programs. These organizations go by a variety of names, such as professional associations or professional societies, etc.

Importance of Professional Organization

❖ Ensuring the credibility of the professional activities.
❖ Ensuring the quality and standards based on the changing trends in the health care system.
❖ Helps in the professional advancement of the members of the profession by organizing continuing educational programs.

■ INTERNATIONAL PROFESSIONAL ORGANIZATIONS

There are many international professional nursing organization, some of these are discussed in this chapter, such as International Council of Nursing (ICN), International Confederation of Midwives (ICM) and International Federation of Perioperative Nurses (IFPN), etc.

International Council of Nurses (ICN)

The International Council of Nurses is a non-political, self-governing federation of national nurse associations dedicated to improving nursing service and education standards, growing nursing as a profession, and maintaining the socioeconomic well-being of nurses in their native countries. ICN is the oldest worldwide professional association in the field of healthcare, having been founded in 1899. The headquarter of ICN is in Geneva, Switzerland.

Mission

To advance nursing as a profession and influence health policy on a global scale.

Activities

Coordination with other international organizations in the health care profession and acting as a voice for nurses on an international level are significant aspects of the ICN's work.

Objectives of ICN

- To encourage the formation of a strong national organization of nurses
- To support the National Nurses Association in improving nursing standards and nurse competency
- To help national nurse organizations in improving the standing of nurses in their respective nations
- To be the world's most authoritative voice for nurses and nursing

Functions of ICN

- ❖ To give policy direction to achieve ICN's goals.
- ❖ To define membership classifications and their rights and responsibilities.
- ❖ To act on the board of directors' recommendations regarding the admission and readmission of member associations to the ICN.
- ❖ To receive and consider information about ICN activities from the board.
- ❖ To receive nominations for the board of directors and to elect the board of directors.
- ❖ To vote on proposed changes to the ICN constitution.
- ❖ To implement the ICN board of directors suggestion.
- ❖ To act on ICN business that requires a rapid response by mail or any written correspondence.
- ❖ Official publication of the journal—International Nursing review.

International Confederation of Midwives (ICM)

ICM is a non-profit organization that represents midwives and midwifery to organizations all over the world to achieve common aims in the care of mothers and babies.

Vision

ICM envisions a society in which every childbearing woman and her newborn have access to midwifery care.

Mission

To promote autonomous midwives as the best caregivers for childbearing women and to maintain birth normal to improve the procreative health of women, their babies, and their families, as well as to create Midwives' Associations and progress the profession of midwifery globally.

International Federation of Perioperative Nurses (IFPN)

The IFPN is a non-profit organization dedicated to the development of perioperative nursing globally. This organization works to assist perioperative nurses around the world in their activities to reform patient outcomes by advocating a secure surgical environment through evidence-based, high-quality researched practice and skills training, in partnership with member organizations and other appropriate collaborators.

Vision

To promote perioperative nursing on a worldwide scale.

■ INDIAN PROFESSIONAL NURSING ORGANIZATIONS

Trained Nurses' Association of India (TNAI), Student Nurses' Association of India (SNAI), Nurses League of Christian Medical Association of India and Indian Society of Psychiatric Nurses (ISPN) are some of the important national nursing organisations, which are discussed in this chapter.

Trained Nurses' Association of India (TNAI)

The Trained Nurses' Association of India (TNAI) is a nationwide body that manages all levels of nurse practitioners. When it was founded in 1908, it was known as the Association of Nursing Superintendents.

Objectives

- To maintain the nursing profession's dignity and honor in every way
- To foster among nurses a strong sense of esprit de corps
- To promote the professional, academic, financial, and overall health of nurses

Functions

- Establishing nursing education standards and putting them in place through suitable routes.
- Establishing nursing service standards and putting them in place through suitable means.
- To create an ethical code of behavior for practitioners.
- Encouraging and promoting research aimed at expanding knowledge to improve evidence-based nursing practice.
- Regarding legislative action, promote legislation and advocate on behalf of nurses.
- Promoting and preserving nurses' financial well-being.
- Offering nurses expert placement and counseling services.
- Making sure that practitioners' professional development is ongoing.
- Speaking to relevant national and international organizations, government agencies, other associations, and the general public on behalf of nurses.
- Providing care following the changing demands of society.

Student Nurses' Association of India (SNAI)

Student nurses in India are represented by the Student Nurses' Association of India (SNAI), which is an allied association that functions under the aegis of TNAI. The fundamental goal of SNAI was to preserve the dignity of students with professional ethics and to foster a sense of community among them. SNAI was founded in Madras during the TNAI Annual Conference in 1929.

Objectives

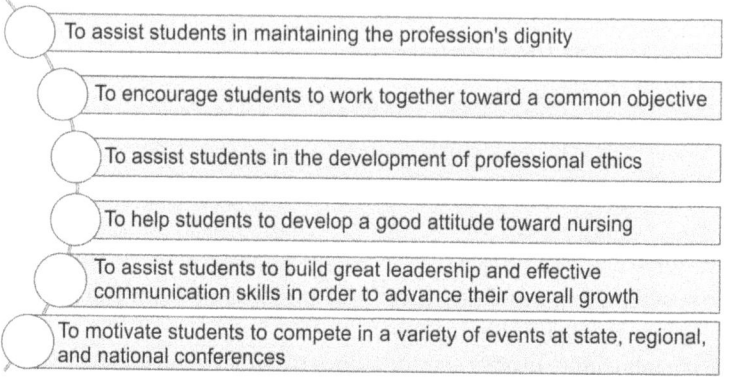

Activities of SNAI

The key activities of the Student Nurses' Association of India (SNAI) are illustrated in **Fig. 3.3**.

Indian Society of Psychiatric Nurses (ISPN)

Under the Societies Act, the International Society of Mental Health Nursing and Allied Health Professionals (ISPN) is a recognized society of Mental Health Nursing and Allied Health Professionals. The mission of this organization is to develop professional and scientific

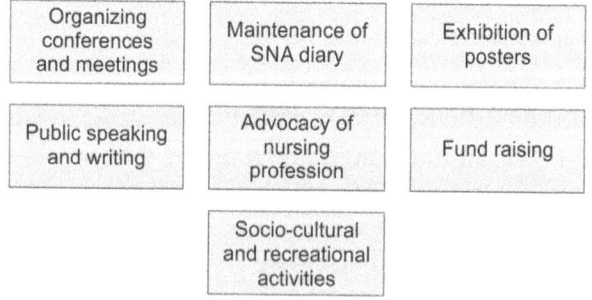

Fig. 3.3: Key activities of the SNAI.

knowledge in the field of mental health nursing. ISPN began in 1991 at NIMHANS. Vision:
- ❖ To provide a venue for conversation and exchange of notions on evidence-based practice in the field of psychiatric nursing, as well as to increase advanced knowledge and skills in the field.
- ❖ Raising awareness and putting study findings into practice.
- ❖ Promote a professional team and collaboration among psychiatric nurses as member of this professional association.

■ CHAPTER HIGHLIGHTS

- ❖ A regulatory body is a formal institution, established by statute or by an authorized government agency that implements the regulatory process as a means of bringing order, uniformity, and control to a profession and its practice.
- ❖ A professional organization is also known as a professional association or professional body.
- ❖ A professional organization is in charge of ensuring that the occupation is practiced legally.
- ❖ Different international and national professional nursing organizations are exiting and are working to foster the growth of the nursing profession.
- ❖ Currently, India has TNAI, SNAI, the Indian Society of Psychiatric Nurses, and many more organizations to set a higher standard of nursing care.
- ❖ These professional organizations provide membership for the nurses.

■ MULTIPLE CHOICE QUESTIONS

1. In which year Indian Nursing Council established?
    a. 1945   b. 1946
    c. 1947   d. 1948
2. In which year international council of nurses established?
    a. 1887   b. 1888
    c. 1889   d. 1899
3. In which year Indian society for psychiatric nurses established?
    a. 1989   b. 1990
    c. 1991   d. 1992

4. In which year trained nurses' association of India (TNAI) established?
   a. 1905
   b. 1906
   c. 1907
   d. 1908
5. In which year student nurses' association of India established?
   a. 1909
   b. 1919
   c. 1929
   d. 1939

ANSWERS

1. c   2. d   3. c   4. d   5. c

BIBLIOGRAPHY

1. Indian Nursing Council. Available from https://www.indiannursingcouncil.org/
2. Indian Society of Psychiatric Nurses (ISPN). Available from https://ispnindia.org/
3. International Confederation of Midwives. Available from https://internationalmidwives.org/about-us/international-confederation-of-midwives/
4. International Council of Nurses. Available from https://www.icn.ch/
5. International Federation of Perioperative Nurses (IFPN). Available from https://www.ifpn.world/
6. Nair S, Healey M. A profession on the margins: Status issues in Indian nursing. Available from http://hdl.handle.net/2451/34246
7. Tiwari RR, Sharma K, Zodpey SP. Situational analysis of nursing education and work force in India, Nursing outlook. 2013 May 1;61(3);129-36.
8. Trained Nurses Association of India (TNAI). Available from https://www.tnaionline.org/

UNIT 2

Professional Values

CHAPTER 4

Professional Values

Suvashri Sasmal, Rakhi Gaur

Learning Objectives

Upon completion of this chapter, the readers should be able to:
- Define personal and professional values in nursing.
- Discuss need for professional values in the nursing profession.
- Explain about professional socialization.
- Describe the importance of professional values in nursing and health care

■ PROFESSIONAL VALUES

Values are the way one thinks, feel acts (makes decisions) in day-to-day life. It is very difficult to define value in a particular way. These are more than ethics, morals, and virtues. It is the foundation of perception that leads the action of an individual that reflects his or her identity as a member of various social groups such as family and organization. In short values are the *"guiding principles of an individual."*

Values are beliefs and goals that guide behavior and serve as a foundation for decision-making. Values provide a framework for evaluating behavior. Nursing is a profession that is grounded in many core values such as altruism, autonomy, the dignity of human beings, integrity, honesty, social justice, and fairness. These core values reflect the spiritual and human approach to nursing and are shared by the entire global community. The values of patient care are affected by the cultural, religious, and economic conditions in each country.

Ethical codes reflect professional values. The code of ethics is designed to help nurses understand the nature of their profession, how they should be treated, and what professional standards they must adhere to nursing, it is becoming more important to promote professional values due to the complexity and increasing number of ethical dilemmas in care settings. To promote the nursing profession, values must be acquired and internalized. They will guide practice and become the standard for nursing. To ensure the future success of nursing, it is important to integrate professional values into nursing education.

Definitions

- According to M. Haralambos, "a value is a belief that something is good and desirable".
- According to R.K. Mukherjee, "values are socially approved desires and goals that are internalized through the process of conditioning, learning or socialization and that become subjective preferences, standards, and aspirations."
- According to Zaleznik and David, "values are the ideas in the mind of men compared to norms in that they specify how people should behave. Values also attach degrees of goodness to activities and relationships."
- Values are defined by Schwartz (1994) as "guiding principles in the life of a person that motivates action, function as standards for judging and justifying action, and that is acquired both through socialization and through the unique learning experiences."

Characteristics of Values

- Values represent an individual's highest priorities based on their deeply held driving forces.
- Values are the powerful forces that affect behavior and personality of an individual.
- Values contain a judgment element, which helps to decide between right and wrong.
- Values are imparted by family, educational institutions, society and peer groups, religion/culture, media, and environment.
- Many values (innate or acquired) are relatively constant and durable.
- Values, norms, and ethics are interrelated concepts with a very fine difference between them.
- Values are fairly permanent, stable, and long-lasting.

Types of Values

Values vary from person to person and some of the basic types of values are mentioned here.

- ❖ **Positive and negative values:** Desirable behavior which is socially acceptable is known as positive values. The exact opposite one is understood as negative values.
- ❖ **Dominant and variant values:** Dominant value is the behavior that cannot be violated in society, e.g., nonviolence. Variant values are the values in which an individual can make a choice, e.g. vegetarian or nonvegetarian.
- ❖ **Innate and acquired values:** Innate values are governed by genes and conscience whereas acquired values are imparted by social institutions such as family, school, and peer group.
- ❖ **Intrinsic and extrinsic values:** Intrinsic values are unique to an individual and are independent of other things. Extrinsic values are the means of achieving intrinsic value, e.g., playing music (extrinsic value) is the means of achieving happiness/inner peace (intrinsic value).

Value Clarification

Value clarification is the process of identifying and examining one's values and systems. There are many steps involved in value clarification. These include "choosing", which is the act of choosing from a variety of options and reflecting on the consequences. "Prizing" means that beliefs are valued and treasured. These beliefs are valued and treasured. "Acting" is incorporating them into your life and behavior. These steps will help in identifying personal values **(Fig. 4.1)**.

Values clarification refers to a process by which individuals can identify, evaluate, and develop their values. Raths Harmin and Simon called it a "valuing procedure:"

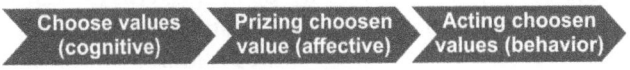

Fig. 4.1: Process of value clarification.

Strategies for Value Clarification

There are numerous strategies used for value clarification. The following are the brief description of strategies that can be used for value clarification relevant to the nursing discipline.

a. **The strategy I—name tag:** Take a piece of paper and write down the name of the nurse in the middle. In the four corners of the paper, write the answer to the following questions.
   - What two things you would like to hear from your colleagues to say about you?
   - The most important thing you will do to improve the nurse-patient interaction
   - What do you do daily to value your health?
   - What are the three values that are most important to you?

   Once the answers are ready one must look into the matter and find out whether they felt any difficulty in answering the questions or if they identified another interlinked question that needs to be answered. In this way, one can reach their value clarification.

b. **Strategy II, Patterns:** In this strategy, an individual identifies their patterns and also reflects whether they require any improvement or alteration in the pattern or not.

   > The following are some of the patterns of values. Underline some of these values you feel most accurately describe you as a professional person. Try to answer some questions for a personal reflection of your values.
   >
   > **Ambitious, reserved, assertive, easily hurt, outgoing, generous, independent, reliable, self-controlled, suspicious, capable, indifferent, dependent, fun-loving, obedient, self-discipline, helpful, moody, imaginative, emotional, affectionate, compromising, argumentative, and solitary**
   >
   > 1. Are you happy with your patterns of values?
   > 2. Do you choose to change the patterns of values you have? Why?
   > 3. List some goals for life-based on the pasterns of values.
   > 4. What patterns do you feel a nurse should ideally possess?
   >
   > *Adapted from Diane B. Uustal (1978)*

c. **Forced choice rank**
   In this method, an imaginary situation and a list of probable reactions are given to the individual from which the individual has

to choose his/her probable reaction. Once the reaction is chosen; the individual is asked to affirm the choice and explain why he/she might feel in that particular way and what might be the pros and cons of the reaction and the value clarification is achieved with the preceding question.

E.g. With whom among your students, you will get most angry? The student
- Who never submits assignments timely
- Who refuses to work with a comatose patient in the ward.
- Rarely helps others or participates least in group projects.

d. **Values continuum:** In this method, the individual is asked a series of question/a single questions. After careful consideration of the questions, the individual indicates his/her standpoint along with a written explanation.

For example, how do you feel about abortion?

Not appropriate under any circumstances ——— **Neutral** ——— Appropriate as per priority

e. **Values voting:** In this method, a list of positive and negative statements are given and the individual has to answer the responses as strongly agree (SA), agree (A), undecided (U), disagree (D), and strongly disagree (SD)

For example, continuing education in nursing is worthwhile to ensure professional identity? Indicate whether you SA, A, U, D, SD, and why?

f. **Unfinished sentence:** In this method, a sentence is given to the individual and they are asked to finish it on their own. These sentences promote thinking at the individual level.

For example, **I wish my clinical instructor would have**_____
I wonder about _____

g. **Alternative search:** Here, an imaginary situation is given and the individual is asked to solve the situation with possible alternatives that they—(i) will try, (ii) will consider trying it, or (iii) will not consider.

Value Neutrality

It is the ability to care for patients while ignoring personal values. Equality of care and support for every patient is possible by being neutral and nonjudgmental. Trust is built between the patient and nurse by offering unconditional support, listening to, and acknowledging their feelings. Conflicting values almost always lead to ethical dilemmas. It is important to recognize the difference between value, fact, or opinion to resolve ethical dilemmas. People sometimes have strong values and consider the facts. Sometimes, people can be so passionate about their beliefs that they cause conflict by provoking judgmental attitudes. Clarifying the values, whether they are own or those of patients, is an essential part of ethical discourse. Values clarification helps to accept differences and often, although not always, it is the key to solving ethical dilemmas. For instance, some people may prefer to be silent during crises while others express it to others to get support and better understanding.

Value Formation

Each culture has its expressions of the fundamental need to nurture and love children and the formation of values is a process that involves schools, government, religious traditions, as well as other social institutions. As children grow, there will be variations in the way that they are raised. These can reinforce or challenge family values. Individuals acquire values over time by choosing the ones they feel most strongly about and possibly discarding or changing others. Individual experiences, i.e., the adverse events of life, can also influence value formation. One who has suffered a lot in their early years of life may be more likely to value things than someone who has not experienced such loss.

A value is an individual belief about the value of a certain idea or custom. This belief sets standards that can influence behavior. Nursing is a profession that requires intimacy. Nursing calls for an interaction with patients emotionally, spiritually, and psychologically. These values are influenced by cultural and social factors. They change and evolve. The nurses inevitably have to work with patients or colleagues who have different values. Therefore, it is crucial to understand our values and be able to communicate our opinions and values to others. In some cultures, decisions regarding health care are made in a group or family-based discussion and not by an individual. This practice can challenge the commitment to the nursing profession and patient autonomy.

■ Critical Thinking
What are the professional values in nursing that distinguish Indian nurses from Western nurses?

Personal and Professional Values

Personal values are the values that one carries with him or her from the culture and society in which he/she lives. To feel accepted, people, need to be able to identify with their culture and have personal values. The professional values are those acquired through socialization in nursing from codes and ethics, nurse's experiences, and peers.

Personal Values

Personal values are the "broad desirable goals that motivate people's actions and serve as guiding principles in their lives."

The ten most important personal values according to Schwartz's value theory (1992) are described as follows:

1. **Self-direction:** The ability and freedom to cultivate one's ideas and abilities (thoughts) and freedom to determine one's actions. These are reflected in choosing own goals, independent thoughts, creativity, curiosity, and exploring the environment.
2. **Stimulation:** This is the ability to feel the presence of excitement, novelty, and challenge in life which are necessary to enrich the experience of an individual.
3. **Hedonism:** This is the ability to have pleasure, enjoyment, and sensuous gratification for oneself.
4. **Achievement:** This is the ability to succeed while demonstrating socially acceptable competence (being ambitious, capable, influential and successful).
5. **Power:** It is the social status and prestige that one possesses along with dominance upon people and resources (social power, wealth, and authority) while maintaining one's public image and avoiding humiliation.
6. **Security:** This includes safety, harmony, and stability of social relationships, and self. Actions directed toward the personal environment (self, family, friends, and reciprocation of favors) and society at large.
7. **Conformity:** This is the ability to control actions and impulses that are likely to upset or harm others and violate social expectations. A person must be polite, obedient, have self-discipline, and respect for elders.
8. **Tradition:** This is considered as the feeling of respect, commitment, and acceptance of the customs and ideas of traditional culture and religion.

9. **Benevolence:** This is the value that one cultivates for the welfare of the people with whom one is in frequent personal contact. It includes being loyal, responsible, honest, helpful, forgiving reliable, and trustworthy.
10. **Universalism:** It is the ability to understand, appreciate, be tolerant, and protective of the welfare of people and nature.

Professional Values in Nursing

Professional nursing values are defined as important professional nursing principles of human dignity, integrity, altruism, and justice that serve as a framework for standards, professional practice, and evaluation. —*Bonnie J Schmidt, 2018*

Some of the professional values relevant to nursing are discussed here.

- ❖ **Human dignity means** giving respect to individuals. It includes respecting persons, their families, and the sociocultural background of the patient. Society has been mentioned as an important nursing ethical value. In nursing, respecting human dignity is consideration of human's innate values, respecting patient's beliefs and preservation of their dignity and privacy during clinical procedures, communicating with the patients with due respect, understanding the patients, and devotion to fulfilling clients' needs. For example, in a clinical setting, the nurse must call the patient with due respect by name instead of calling them "uncle" or "aunty".
- ❖ **Social justice** is the fair distribution of resources and provision of equal treatment and cares to individuals irrespective of economic, social, and cultural status.
- ❖ **Altruism** means the spirit of selflessness and helpfulness toward others. In this value, humans are the axis of attention. It denotes, helping others, making provision of the utmost health and welfare for the clients, their families, and society, selflessly with self-devotion.
- ❖ **Autonomy in decision making:** This means the right of independence in decision making, the right to accept or reject suggested treatments, interventions, or care. Nurses must help the client in decision-making by giving appropriate and adequate information to the clients and, to their families when necessary.
- ❖ **Precision and accuracy in caring** are indicated as the most important nursing value. Nursing care should be based on a sound

standard of practice which must be precise, safe, appropriate, multidimensional, kind, and satisfying. The care must be safe enough to promote their health and relieve their pain and suffering.

- ❖ **Responsibility** is defined as the commitment to giving evidence-based care, being responsible toward patients, and respecting the patient's rights in decision-making.
- ❖ **A human relationship** is the ability of the nurse to maintain honesty in words and practice, be sympathetic, and have mutual understanding, courtesy, and friendliness with clients. Standard of practice in patient care is possible when humanistic, efficient, and effective relationships, a relationship is made with clients.
- ❖ **Individual and professional competency** is defined as the traits of struggling to make nursing a profession, feeling the need to acquire personal and professional competency in the direction of adaptation of new technology and new evidence. Personal and professional competency is usually achieved by lifelong learning, participating in continuing education, research, and quality control activities.
- ❖ **Sympathy** is the trait of understanding patients' and their families' needs and giving care based on making fair communication. Empathy is an integral part of sympathy. It is characterized by nurse's ability to understand the feeling, experiences, or psychosocial abilities of their patients by placing themselves in their situation.
- ❖ **Trust** is the trait of honesty in words and practice. Nurses should gain patient's, their families,' and society's trust through understanding patient's situation and status and appropriate conformation with them.

■ PROFESSIONAL SOCIALIZATION: INTEGRATION OF PROFESSIONAL VALUES WITH PERSONAL VALUES

The term "socialization" describes the process through which people acquire the knowledge, abilities, and attitudes needed for them to be able to contribute to their community. Learning about one's self-concept, subcultures, and family roles and norms is the first step in socialization. People can develop their self-concept by joining new groups as they get older and take on new roles, learn new norms, and do so.

People who wish to be a professional must undergo professional socialization. Professional socialization refers to the process of becoming a legitimate member of a professional organization.

This idea was relatively obscure until the 1940s, but after World War II, it caught the attention of numerous academics and philosophers across many fields, and it was added to dictionaries. Professional socialization is the essence of a successful academic experience. Any dissatisfaction or distressing experience might lead to a pupil dropping out of the institution and the profession itself. The proper understanding of personal values increases the awareness of professional values which will eventually reflect professionalism. The pioneer of the nursing profession, Florence Nightingale emphasized character development and professional socialization during the training period to ensure the successful transition from a student nurse to a professional nurse.

The journey to professional socialization looks like an adventure that takes the person from being marginal to fully participate in a professional society. However, professional socialization is not the same as mere education. In any profession, training is the process of learning new information and skills. Socialization is the combination of this knowledge with a new sense of self. For a successful academic experience, professional socialization is vital. Thus professional socialization is a process to acquire specialized knowledge, skills, attitudes, values, norms, and interests within nursing.

Definition

- ❖ "Professional socialization is defined as the knowledge and skill that characteristics of a profession" (Becker-Hentz, 2005).
- ❖ "Professional socialization is a process through which a person acquires the knowledge, skills, values and ethical standards to form a professional identity." (Hao, Niu, Li, Yue, and Liu, 2014).

Importance of Professional Socialization

- ❖ Promotes effective communication with patients and healthcare team members.
- ❖ Increases self-awareness leading to self-development in terms of development of character and personality.

- ❖ Improves participation, performance, and job satisfaction which leads to retention within the profession.
- ❖ Helps in resolving role conflicts as they adopt and adapt to professional roles
- ❖ Enhances behavioral and professional commitment
- ❖ Helps in the identification of the philosophy of the profession and motivates career progression

Factors Affecting Professional Socialization

a. *Professional factors*
   - Difference between theory and practice in terms of application of knowledge and skills.
   - Tacit knowledge gained through communication within the group.
   - Discrimination and isolation based on educational qualification and years of experience.
   - Quality and support of the administrators.
b. *Personal factors*
   - Personal sociocultural context and beliefs
   - Coping ability and adaptability
   - The ability of time management
   - Educational experiences
   - Choice of defense mechanism
   - Openness to others, communication patterns specifically social interaction pattern
   - The practice of reflection and role observation
   - Ability to maintain balance
   - Desire to update professional knowledge
   - Internal motivation for forming professional identity
c. *Educational factors*
   - Student-teacher relationships such as interaction patterns and a supportive environment
   - Curricular pattern
   - Extracurricular activities
   - Resilience to maintain professional ideals
   - Years of education and experience

Ineffective professional socialization can have various negative impacts on nurses which are as follows:
- Demoralization and poor performance leading to low quality of service
- Reduced productivity
- Nonacceptance of the role leads to frequent job changes
- Lack of interest and leaving the organization or profession
- Negative body image and psychological stress

Measures to Promote Professional Socialization in Nursing Educational Setting

To encourage professional socialization in nursing, the following actions must be taken:
- Orientation of students must be done on exposure to a new clinical area.
- Genuine interest and involvement in student's professional life by comprehending their educational and instructional requirements, and acting accordingly.
- Maintain a positive and growing relationship with students'
- Appreciate the contribution of students to the interdisciplinary team.
- Working together with clinical nurses to support students in integrating theory and practice by fostering discussion and implementing reflective exercises.
- Provide students with constructive criticism and guidance as they develop appropriate behavior.
- Encouraging dialog and initiating brainstorming activities, role-playing, simulation, and supervised clinical observation sessions which must be followed by a reflective learning exercise for understanding the unpredictable clinical environments.
- Emphasis on competency development, while taking into account learning objectives, the minimum number of hours required, and available clinical facilities.
- Ensure meaningful learning opportunities for the students'
- Regular communication about issues involving students with the appropriate stakeholders.
- Avoid all measures of inequalities such as gender, religion, and caste biases.

❖ Have access to counseling services for students whenever necessary.
❖ Create awareness of the various legislative measures among students to avoid violation of ethical principles.
❖ Monitor students for any misconduct and follow the standard guidelines for dealing with misconduct rather than personal judgment.
❖ Create a positive learning environment where everyone is treated with dignity which will help students to identify an ideal work environment.

Integration of Professional Values with Personal Values

Integration of professional and personal values occurs with the interplay of various factors. Philip J. Osteen published the following model in 2013, which helps to clearly understand how this integration occurs **(Fig. 4.2)**.

According to this model, the integration of personal and professional values has three distinct but related components—

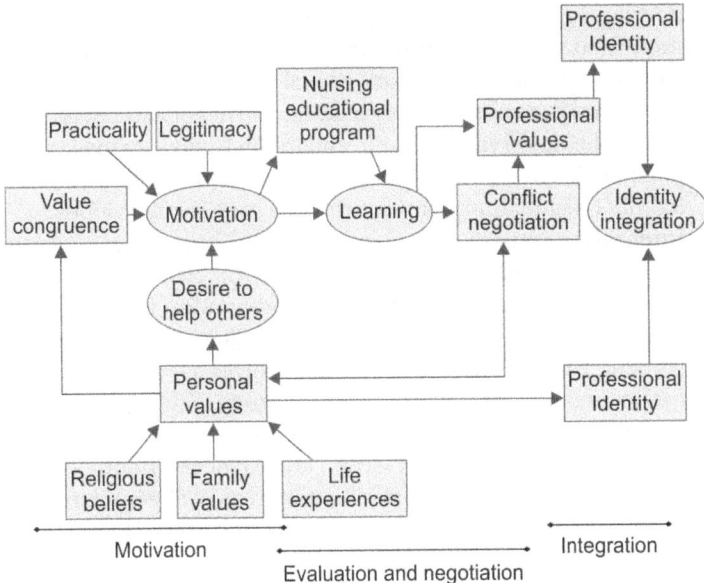

Fig. 4.2: Model of integration of professional values with personal values.
Source: Adapted from Philip J. Osteen (2013).

(1) motivation, (2) evaluation and negotiation, and (3) integration.
1. **Motivation** is denoted on the left-hand side of the model, which illustrates the different types of motivators that influenced student's decisions to enter a professional educational program such as nursing. These motivational factors are mentioned here.
   - **Personal values** are influenced by *family values* (in which a person grows up) *religious beliefs* (belief in the supreme power) and the day-to-day *life experiences* that a person gathers.
   - **Desire to help others** stem from the personal values which motivate a person to pursue a carrier in nursing or other professional courses.
   - **Value congruence** explains the reason behind a person's willingness to follow rules, regulations, and values. It refers to the extent to which the personal values of a person are as per the surroundings.
   - **Practicality and legitimacy are the motivational factors denoting the desire for** being successful in life and focusing on acquiring the skills and knowledge to practice competently.
2. **Evaluation and negotiation** are the second components of the integration of personal and professional values which usually develop with the learning experiences of the nursing program. A motivated student is self-directed to gather knowledge and skills which are provided in the professional curriculum. Further, he/she goes through a continuous evaluation and negotiation of personal and professional values. Any in congruence between these values must be discussed or negotiated with their professional mentors (conflict negotiation) for nurturing the professional values.
3. **Integration** consists of the synthesis of personal and professional identities based on the outcomes of the evaluation of their professional values. The process of integration occurs in three stages namely—(1)integrated, (2) nonintegrated, and (3) evolving. Nursing students who mention themselves as "nurse" in social gatherings are at the "integrated" stage. Students who feel uncomfortable expressing themselves under the label of "nurse" to describe their professional selves can be labeled "nonintegrated". This can happen with practicing nurses as well who manage to express themselves as "teachers" only in society rather than "a nursing teacher/a nursing faculty". "Evolving" applies to those students who gladly express themselves as "student nurses" in society. Personal and professional value integration aims to reach the "integrated" stage.

PROFESSIONAL VALUES IN NURSING

Importance of Professional Values in Nursing and Health Care

Values are the guiding principle of personal and professional life. The following list of factors highlights the significance of professional values in nursing and healthcare **(Fig. 4.3)**:

- Professional values help in decision-making in the clinical or community setting.
- It helps in understanding nurse's behavior and its modification as per the requirement.
- It improves understanding of the client and his or her surroundings. This develops a healthy interpersonal relationship between nurses and clients, nurses, and stakeholders involved in healthcare settings.
- Understanding professional values lead to the maintenance of standard nursing care, leading to improved patient satisfaction.
- Increases job satisfaction among nurses and prevents drop out, and migration of nurses.
- Motivates nurses to engage themselves in activities related to continuing education, research, and quality assurance. These ultimately refine the knowledge base of the nursing profession.
- Reduces health care costs by promoting early healing and making people knowledgeable about their health.
- Increases the trust of society toward the nursing profession.

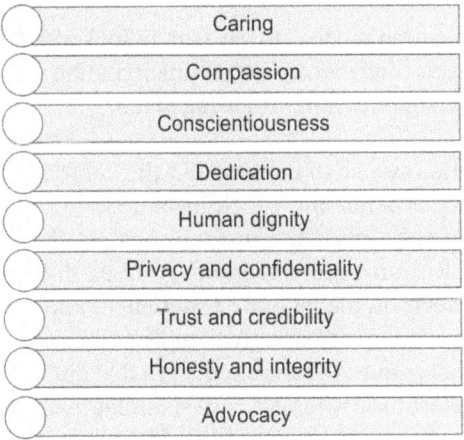

Fig. 4.3: Professional values in nursing.

One of the most respected professions, nursing is founded on moral principles. Human dignity, integrity, compassion, and fairness are significant professional nursing principles that provide a foundation for standards, professional practice, and evaluation. The code of ethics articulates professional principles. Every newly licensed nurse in India is required to abide by the code of ethics and professional conduct for nurses established by the Indian Nursing Council. Some of the important professional values are discussed here:

■ CARING: DEFINITION AND PROCESS

Caring is a universal human nature that promotes a sense of well-being and supports health. It is a unique underlying principle of nursing. Caring is a relationship between nurse and patient based on protection and support for the best interests of the patient. Caring means feeling or showing concern for or kindness to others. It is an expression of respect and cares for others, as demonstrated by one's actions. Various researchers have mentioned caring differently making it difficult to define.

❖ Human caring involves values, a will, and a commitment to care, knowledge, caring actions, and consequences. All of human caring is related to intersubjective human response to health-illness, environmental-personal interaction, knowledge of the nurse caring process; self-knowledge, knowledge of one's power, and transaction limitations."

—Jean Watson

❖ The word caring means "to care for, to look after." It is a natural characteristic of all mankind. This phenomenon is associated with assistance, support, and the easing of life.

—Kutnohorská, 2007

❖ "Care is the essence of nursing and the central, dominant, and unifying focus of nursing" – Leininger, 1991

Caring must be person-centered, protect the patient's best interests, involve nursing interventions, and have the potential to have a variety of effects on the patient's experiences and well-being. As a result of the patient's increasingly complex care needs and the lack of available time, there is a serious concern that nursing practice may become more technical without a corresponding increase in the caring component. Nurses who are focused on the human relationship must see, understand, and accept responsibility to provide care. It is critical to emphasize caring concepts in nursing because they can help nurses better reflect on their moral principles and advance their knowledge of caring in nursing practice. According to Florence Nightingale, the purpose of nursing is to place the patient in the optimal environment to allow nature to take its course. According to her, the term "nursing" carries some ambiguity and has several meanings. "Nursing" refers to both the care that people provide to one another and the care that those in need of assistance get. Nursing was seen as a practice that promoted health and well-being and allowed patients to utilize their resources as much as possible.

Characteristics of Caring

- Caring takes place every time, when the nurse-to-patient contact is made.
- It is essential to nursing because it helps nurses get close to patients
- Caring may occur without curing but curing cannot occur without caring (Watson 2003).
- The one caring and the one being cared for are interconnected. It is a deeper level of human connection than a physical interaction (Watson 1997).
- It is the emotional support that gives patients a sense of peace or security in hospital settings.
- Caring means tending, playing, and learning, which can generate trust, meet the patient's needs, provide physical and spiritual well-being and create a feeling of being in development to support the health processes (Eriksson, 1997).
- It alleviates the patient's suffering by enabling the best possible medical treatment.
- Caring requires the spiritual, moral, personal, and social engagement of a nurse with a commitment to self and other community.

Components of Caring

Caring has two fundamental components which are listed here:
1. *The technical and physical component*: This is the act of caring such as assisting, helping, and serving which are mediated through the nurse-patient relationship.

2. *The psychological and emotional component*: This includes the "attitudes and feelings" aspect of caring in which the nurse understands the patient and acts accordingly.

Apart from these fundamental components, the "five C's of caring" provide additional meaning to the concept of caring. The following are as described by Sister Simone Roach **(Fig. 4.4)**.

- ❖ **Commitment:** The life of a nurse can be difficult at times, but there are a lot of different ways to show your dedication to the profession. It may take the form of a commitment to patients, coworkers, or employers, in addition to a commitment to one's health and life outside of work.
- ❖ **Compassionate care:** Care should be provided not only because it is required, but also to provide compassionate care that extends beyond meeting physical needs to meet emotional ones as well.
- ❖ **Courageousness:** Nurses need the courage to care for their patients who may have various illnesses including infectious diseases. They must show courage by offering comfort and hope during adverse events of the treatment process and find their strength within themselves.
- ❖ **Competence:** Numerous methods exist for nurses to demonstrate their competence. Nurses can demonstrate their competence by

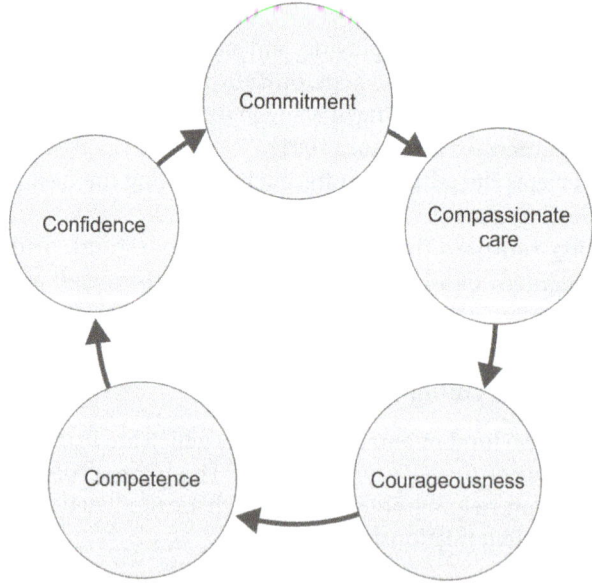

Fig. 4.4: Five C's of caring.

rendering their practice with professional skills. In addition, nurses can collaborate with other healthcare team members to provide patient-centered care of the highest quality.
- **Confidence:** Confidence is the aspect of caring that connects everything, and it is not limited to the nurse. To provide care for a patient, nurses must be confident in their abilities, which will also energize the patient.

Importance of Caring Behavior

Various nurse researchers have reported the following findings related to caring in their studies which reflect the importance of caring in nursing:
- Enhances the patient's ability for faster healing.
- Improves patients' understanding of their health and wellness, and builds up the confidence.
- Increases voluntary patient participation and cooperation in health care activities.
- Decreases mortality rates and hospitalization rates, and reduces healthcare costs.

The Caring Behavior and the Nursing Practice

The nurses can demonstrate caring behavior in many ways. **Table 4.1** summarizes some of the behaviors through which the nurses can express caring while delivering their practice.

Table 4.1: Caring behavior during nursing care.
- Smiling face
- Making eye contact
- Greeting and calling the patient by their name instead of bed number
- Active listening without interrupting
- Use therapeutic touch
- Avoid being judgmental
- Comforting patients as per requirement
- Answer the questions therapeutically
- Supporting in activities of daily living (such as bathing and walking)
- Showing patience as per the needs
- Being responsible and assisting in clinical decision-making
- Respecting patients and families irrespective of their healthcare choices

■ COMPASSION: SYMPATHY VERSUS EMPATHY AND ALTRUISM

Compassion, sympathy, empathy, and altruism are interrelated concepts in nursing. They are often used interchangeably within healthcare policy, delivery, and research in describing some of the human qualities that patients desire in their healthcare providers.

- ❖ Sympathy is "the verbal and nonverbal expression of sorrow or concern" (Morse et al, 1992).
- ❖ Compassion is " active participation in another individual's suffering" (Schantz, 2007).
- ❖ Empathy is "the ability to understand and share the feelings of another." Someone can put himself in another's shoes and feel what that person is going through and share their emotions and feelings. They share elements with other forms of prosocial behavior such as generosity, kindness, and patient-centeredness Empathy "allows understanding not only of other's beliefs, values, and ideas but also the significance that their situation has for them and their associated feelings" (Rogers, 1951).

Compassion

Compassion is a word with Latin roots that means "to suffer with." It means "to share in the suffering of another." It is considered the feeling when we confront suffering and are motivated to alleviate that suffering. Nursing places high importance on compassion since it makes patients feel appreciated while receiving medical treatment. Compassion can be demonstrated in various ways such as paying attention to patient's worries, responding to those worries right away, and using compassionate language while delivering treatments. This is considered by many nurses to be one of the essential elements of high-quality treatment.

Sympathy versus Empathy

- ❖ Sympathy is defined as an expression of concern for other's misfortune, especially when they are perceived to be suffering unjustly. Empathy, on the other hand, has been defined as the capacity to comprehend and accurately acknowledge the emotions of another and therapeutically act on them.

- ❖ In comparison to sympathy, empathy is a more expansive and strenuous emotional response.
- ❖ An empathetic relationship encourages the sharing of innermost feelings. It is the feeling of a situation someone else is going through.
- ❖ Nurses who are sympathetic feelings toward the patient, while nurses who are empathetic feel for the patient. As a result, when a nurse empathizes, they share some of the emotion and feeling of the person they are helping.
- ❖ A person's ability to empathize is influenced by prior exposure to a similar situation.

Components of Empathy

Some of the integral components of empathy are listed below **(Fig. 4.5)**.

- ❖ **Cognitive empathy:** Cognitive empathy is the ability to identify and understand another person's feelings and perspective from an objective stance. It is the detached acknowledgment and understanding of a distressing situation based on someone's sense of duty. This aspect of empathy truly differentiates empathy from sympathy and compassion.

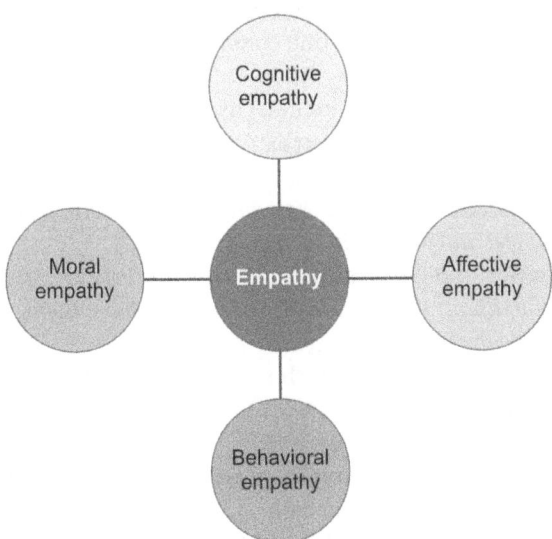

Fig. 4.5: Components of empathy.

- ❖ **Affective empathy**: It is the ability to subjectively experience and shares in another psychological state or feelings. It is all of the elements of cognitive empathy plus acknowledgment and understanding of someone's situation by "feeling with" him.
- ❖ **Behavioral empathy**: This is communicating the understanding with the patient and acting out to reduce the distress of the patient.
- ❖ **Moral empathy**: This is an internal motivation of concern for the other and a desire to act to relieve their suffering by caring and driving acts of altruism.

Benefits from Sympathetic and Empathetic Nursing Practices

- ❖ It helps to lower physical and psychological distress.
- ❖ It helps to improve client satisfaction and positive feedback on nursing care.
- ❖ Increased client compliance leads to positive health outcomes.
- ❖ Improves competency and enhances job satisfaction.
- ❖ Helps to reduce malpractice.

Strategies to Provide Sympathetic and Empathetic Nursing Care

- ❖ Listen to patients carefully and acknowledge their feelings
- ❖ Give attention to nonverbal cues.
- ❖ Being empathetic. The nurse can express empathy by using judiciously using therapeutic communication techniques in the following ways.
  - **N**ame or mirror the emotion (Ex: "*You seem very stressed.*")
  - **U**nderstand the emotion (Ex: "*It can be stressful to wait for your blood tests when it's about your health.*")
  - **R**espect the client (Ex: "*You did a great job with telling us how you feel and coming here to do these tests.*")
  - **S**upport the client using powerful words (Ex: "*I will let you know about your results as soon as we have them, and we'll decide the next steps together.*")
  - **E**xplore the emotion further (Ex: "*Is there something else on your mind that bothers you?*")
- ❖ Be friendly, kind, and respectful.
- ❖ Be aware of the sociocultural context of the patient's problem and adapt culturally congruent care.
- ❖ Use self-relaxation and reflective strategies to avoid mental agony.

Altruism

The word altruism is derived from the Latin *letter huic*, which means selfless concern for the well-being of others. Altruism is depicted as the heart of nursing. The altruistic behavior of the nurses is socially directed to relieve difficulties, problems, and pain associated with patients. The profession has been characterized by self-professed altruism which means, a selfless service on behalf of or for others. According to Henderson, "the primary and unique task of the nurse is to help healthy or sick individuals to maintain their health or to die during their treatment or in peace." Empathy motivates altruistic behavior.

Type of Altruism

There are several different types of altruistic behavior. These include **genetic altruism** (altruistic acts for the benefit of close family members), **reciprocal altruism** (engagement in altruistic behavior to get favor in return), **group-selected altruism** (efforts are directed toward helping people of a social group from where future supports can be expected) and **pure altruism**. Nurses work with pure altruism. In this form, people are motivated by internalized values and morals. Nurses help someone else, even when it is risky, without zeal for rewards (e.g., active participation in patient care even if they are in the situation of war, or earthquake).

Characteristics of Altruistic Behaviors

- Open-minded: Ability to view and accept alternative perspectives.
- Awareness of consequences: They have awareness of the consequences of their actions and have the ability to gladly accept them.
- Awareness of self and others.
- Adjustability: Ability to adapt and adjust in any situation transcending the ego.
- Confidence and forgiveness are their core characteristics.
- Proactive in nature: Takes actions of their own.
- Feeling of self-worth by helping others.
- They worry about how their actions might be felt by others

Factors Affecting Altruism

The following factors might have some effect on a nurse's altruistic behavior:

- **Age:** As experiences are gathered over time, older nurses tend to be more empathetic. But sometimes, years of experience adversely affect empathy, as repeated exposure to stressful situations in the clinical field might also make nurses lack altruistic behavior.
- **Gender:** Traditionally, females tend to be more empathetic. However, it is not always true; it might vary with the individual.
- **Work atmosphere:** Congenial environment at the workplace such as adequate nurse-patient ratio and a positive appraisal from patients, coworkers, and organization has a positive impact on developing altruistic behavior.

Benefits of Maintaining Altruistic Behavior

- Altruistic emotions and behaviors are reported to be associated with greater well-being, health, and longevity.
- Increased social support as "doing good to others bring back good".
- Brings spiritual happiness.

Drawbacks of Altruism

- Researchers have found that altruism created a sense of ambivalence and ambiguity among nurses, as they want to respond to "the other's" need, but are also unwilling to take unconditional responsibility for "the other."
- Burnout and psychological distress among nurses.

■ CONSCIENTIOUSNESS

The Oxford dictionary meaning of conscientiousness is, "taking care to do things carefully and correctly." In 1993, psychologist Goldberg introduced the "Big Five Personality Dimensions." It defines most of the personality aspects of individuals and is widely accepted and adopted. Its five dimensions include extroversion, agreeableness, conscientiousness, neuroticism, and openness. All of these are directly related to the performance of a nurse. Conscientiousness is a personality trait that deals with self-regulation and impulse control. They show a preference for planned rather than spontaneous behavior. Conscientiousness is a key personality trait with many characteristics, including self-control, diligence, responsibility, and reliability. The ability to delay desire and adhere to socially dictated norms for impulse control are all characteristics of conscientiousness.

Characteristics of Conscientiousness in Nursing

- They are goal-orientated specifically oriented to their task.
- Conscientious nurses are goal striving, dependable, and maintain orderliness.
- Prefers to complete assigned work much ahead of time as they stay away from procrastination. They never fail to meet a deadline.
- They are a strict follower of rules and regulations and tend to prefer the classical bookish methods. But this hinders their knowledge acquisition by innovation.
- Nurses with higher conscientiousness tend to give focus on each element of their work. It makes the output accurate and of high quality. This provides patient satisfaction and job satisfaction to the nurse also.
- They tend to be visionary with their forward-thinking tendency. It helps them to be prepared ahead of time.
- They are slow decision-makers. They take time to decide because of a detailed weighing of the pros and cons of each option available to them.
- A nurse with higher conscientiousness might show micromanaging tendencies at work because of their achievement orientation and strict adherence to rules. They might be difficult to please.

The Positive Effects of Being Conscientiousness

- They are valued in the workplace because of their ability to prioritize tasks effectively and being disciplined.
- They execute their jobs to perfection and are guided by a sense of duty toward their organizations, peers, and team members.
- Conscientious nurses tend to suffer less from burnout as they finish their work in time.
- They are positively motivated toward their duty and thus possess a positive attitude towards the situations they encounter in daily practice.
- Conscientious people are the least likely to be counterproductive at work such as bad-mouthing coworkers, sudden sick leaves, and bullying.

❖ Researchers have reported that due to well-planned work patterns of conscientious people they tend to suffer less from health issues (e.g., cognitive disorders) in old age.

The Negative Effects of Being Conscientiousness

There are certain drawbacks if a person becomes extremely conscientious such as:

❖ They tend to be perfectionists and thus do not like other's performance. People working under them might feel uncomfortable due to this.
❖ They barely accept criticism which hinders their scope of improvement.
❖ Being overly rigid in being planned might cause mental diseases such as obsessive-compulsive disorders.
❖ They might struggle to act spontaneously which might affect the unpredictable scenarios in a healthcare setting.
❖ It might affect creativity and innovation.

Measures to Improve Conscientiously

The measures to improve conscientiousness while delivering nursing practice are listed here:

❖ **Be reflective in assessing your conscientiousness.**
   By reflectively asking some questions one can assess their conscience nature. Do you finish your work before others? Do you check it twice before submission and get yourself busy in the next one? Do you give your best in doing the assignment? Is it easy for you to avoid distractions? How do you concentrate on your work?
❖ **Get organized and create realistic goals:** Set achievable realistic goals to avoid undue stress. Organize the work stepwise based on the priority.
❖ **Slow down:** Sometimes learn to take a pause. Have some break. This will help to boost your mental energy and speed of work.
❖ **Cultivate the existing conscientious habit:** Be reliable, organized, and punctual. This will build a positive reputation inside the organization as well as with your colleagues and patients. Having a positive image of self as a healthcare team member builds our confidence, and improves the interpersonal relationship and workplace environment.

- **Develop a strong work ethic:** It includes finishing a task on time, respecting each other, and avoiding personal addresses inside the workplace.
- **Look outward and build relationships with colleagues:** Learn to have a balanced work life and personal life.

DEDICATION/DEVOTION TO WORK

The dictionary meaning of these two words is as follows, **"Devotion"** is great admiration, affection, and love for someone. **"Dedication"** denotes willingly giving a lot of time and energy to something because it is important: Dedication/devotion to work is the principal value of nursing. It refers to being dedicated/devoted to the welfare of mankind whether in health or illness.

Dedication in nursing refers to a sentiment, emotional state, or unwavering commitment that defines the profession's art and core values. It involves providing care out of the goodness of one's heart using all available technical and human resources, going above and beyond one's obligations under organizational and legal rules. This behavior typically occurs without any hope of reward or incentive, which puts one in danger of overlooking own needs.

The Manifestation of Dedication and Devotion in Nursing

A good nurse must possess this behavioral characteristic which might be manifested as internal and external attributes.
- *Internally a nurse must feel* a purpose, pride, and satisfaction with the profession. He/she must have courage, motivation, untiring commitment, show responsibility toward their work, i.e., with clients, and feel absorbed while working.
- *External manifestations* of a dedicated nurse will be seen as listening and paying attention, being considerate to the client's needs, helping, caring, and accompanying them. Focusing on the needs, making priorities, perceiving, adopting, and implementing tactfully. Nurses with dedication tend to perform better which will improve patient satisfaction.

Factors Influencing Dedication/Devotion of Nurses

- *Personal factors* such as younger age, sex, higher education, experience, faith/trust in superpowers and humans, sense of

fairness, tolerance, empathetic nature, moral sensitivity, creativity, communication skills, and positive spiritual and ethical values are largely determined by dedication or devotion.
- ***Interpersonal factors*** include having a healthy relationship with family, peers, coworkers, healthcare team members, and patients.
- ***Job-related factors*** include the tenure of the job and its related security (e.g., permanent or contractual), salary, job control, opportunities for career progression and promotion, reward systems, autonomy, clarity of expectations from higher authority, workload, job satisfaction, good appearance in the organization, self-belief in having the right performance, resources and stressors related to the job, and nursing manpower of an organization.
- **Contextual factors:** This includes environmental and developmental factors. Environmental factors include quality of working life (e.g., social prestige) and organizational features. Developmental factors include opportunities for learning, developing skills through continuing education/in-service education, progressing and growing in the career pathway, and availability of career counseling opportunities.

The Outcomes of Dedication in Nursing

There are both positive and negative outcomes of dedication in nursing. Dedicated nurses are protective of their patients. They strive to preserve and promote the patient's health, improve the perceived quality of care, enhancing a sense of coherence. Thus they improve patient satisfaction and reduce hospital stays by promoting early healing. For nurses, positive consequences of dedication manifest as physical and psychological, and family-related well-being, experiencing a high quality of life, healthy lifestyle choices, job satisfaction, social acceptance, and social recognition, lower stress associated with patient care, feeling motivated, and a sense of pride for pursuing this career. For organizations, dedicated nursing personnel will reduce hospital mortality rates, positive feedback from patients, higher financial profit, satisfaction with organizational policies, increased retention of nurses, and satisfaction at various levels of management.

Drawbacks of Being a Dedicated/Devoted Nurse

Balancing work and personal life is always important for everyone. If nurses become over dedicated/devoted they might suffer from physical and psychological consequences such as physical harm or injury (e.g., urinary tract infection from less intake of water and voluntary retention of urine, leg pain due to long-standing hours), exposure to harmful microorganisms of the job environment and burnout (e.g., repeated exposure to critical patients, deaths, and grieving families), excessive stress, role ambiguity, work challenges, more negative attitude toward the job, parental stress, and family conflict.

■ RESPECT FOR THE PERSON-HUMAN DIGNITY

The concept of human dignity is an important professional and ethical value in nursing practice. It expresses the respect for human individuality and the right of each individual to be treated as a unique human being. In 1948, United Nations have declared Human Rights as "recognition of the inherent dignity and the equal and inalienable rights of all members of the human family is the foundation of freedom, justice, and peace in the world." Human dignity is the basic right of each human irrespective of their health status. In the nursing profession, the concept of human dignity is basic, nebulous, multifaceted, and multidimensional. It entails considering each person as an individual and respecting their uniqueness. Patients as well as all other people must have the utmost respect for human dignity. Understanding respect and competence is a prerequisite for human dignity since it enables the individual to feel respected and to grow, develop, and esteem others.

Aspects of Human Dignity

Respect, self-confidence, self-control and environment control, privacy, and identity are the different aspects under its broad heading.

- ❖ **Respect:** Respect, is an important moral principle of human dignity as per Nurse theorist Parse's human becoming theory. Every person should be respected irrespective of their age, gender, social, economic, or financial status.
- ❖ **Self-confidence:** Nursing activities must be directed toward building self-confidence among patients. They must be nonjudgmental even toward a dying patient.

- **Self-control and environmental control** mean ability to control own behavior, movement, control over own lifestyle, and decisions (e.g., having food of own choice, moving around from one place to another, etc.). Environmental control means controlling own surroundings as per one's requirement (controlling light buttons as per the need).
- **Privacy** denotes the most critical aspect of respecting human dignity. It means keeping the patient's information confidential and sharing it judiciously (e.g., privacy of family problems shared by the patient, sharing the information with the psychologists if indicated). It also includes maintenance of privacy of physical proximity (e.g., covering the patient properly while giving intramuscular injections in an immunization clinic, while giving catheter care, etc.).
- **Identity** means how a person perceives himself or others in the professional setting. Each patient is having some unique family and social roles. An example of maintaining human dignity through identity can be calling a child by his name instead of bed number/someone's child.

Facilitators and Threats of Respect for Human Dignity

Nurses must be dedicated to preserving human dignity in their practice. It is achieved by considering patient's values and beliefs in planning care activities, explaining the activities before implementation, making health care accessible to everyone and informing them about their available choices, establishing an open communication environment, being nonjudgmental, orienting the patient with hospital routines and ward set up on admission, paying attention to dietary preferences, etc.

Threats are the factors that might influence human dignity in patient care and may be patient-related or organizations. A patient with an ongoing pathological process is already in a compromised situation which threatens their dignity. Violation of privacy also occurs if any procedure is carried out without explanation, lack of patient and family members participating in the decision-making process, lack of adequate resources (e.g., insufficient bed strength of hospital in comparison to demand, poor nurse-patient ratio, admission to a filthy environment, nonavailability of important supplies such as linen and blankets).

Maintenance of Human Dignity: Positive and Negative Consequences

Nurses who care for human dignity consider patient's values, beliefs, and cultural diversity while planning and implementing care. Maintenance of human dignity by nurses while caring for patients brings the following positive consequences:

- ❖ They feel respected and worthy in healthcare decision-making.
- ❖ Kindness and affection reflected in nursing care increase patient's satisfaction and promote patient's self-esteem and trust in nurses.
- ❖ Positive coping with health and wellness and active participation of patients and family members in rehabilitation and follow-up services.
- ❖ Reduces healthcare costs as the patient feels they have developed an ability to control their environment and self. They positively modify their lifestyle.

The inability of nurses to maintain the human dignity of their patients leads to spiritual and psychological distress and might provoke suicidal tendencies in depressed patients. Respecting human dignity also entails recognizing each patient's right to privacy and the freedom to select their healthcare providers. As one of the most significant professional principles, the idea of human dignity has been included in ethical dilemmas in the fields of education and nursing practice.

■ PRIVACY AND CONFIDENTIALITY: INCIDENTAL DISCLOSURE

Privacy and confidentiality is an important ethical principle in nursing. It is an important legal obligation that all health professionals must obey. Maintenance of privacy and confidentiality is given importance at an early age in nursing. We all take the oath while entering the profession in the form of "Nightingale pledge" to preserve the privacy of our patients.

"…..I will do all in my power to maintain and elevate the standard of my profession, and will hold in confidence all personal matters committed to my keeping and all family affairs coming to my knowledge in the practice of my calling….."   ***Nightingale pledge***

In simple terms, **Privacy** is a basic human right due to which a person is free from public interference. **Confidentiality** is the duty to ensure that the information gathered through a trusting relationship is kept secret.

Incidental disclosure is a situation in which private information is disclosed despite taking adequate measures for example, in an emergency room a patient looking at the X-ray plate of another patient or overhearing information related to another patient while walking through the corridor. U.S. Department of Health and Human Services has given the following definition, "an incidental use or disclosure is a secondary use or disclosure that cannot reasonably be prevented, is limited in nature, and that occurs as a result of another use or disclosure that is permitted by the rule. However, an incidental use or disclosure is not permitted if it is a by-product of an underlying use or disclosure which violates the privacy rule." The essential components of privacy and confidentiality have been depicted in **Figure 4.6**.

Positive Consequences of Maintaining Privacy and Confidentiality in a Clinical Setting

❖ It helps to develop a trusting relationship with the patient.
❖ It improves patient satisfaction.
❖ Positive feedback from patients improves job satisfaction among nurses.
❖ It improves the standard of the nursing profession as society feels it is reliable.

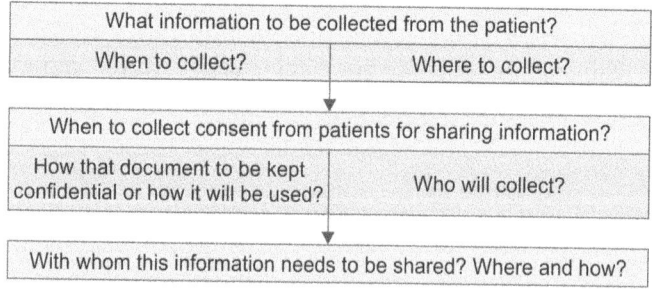

Fig. 4.6: Essential components of privacy and confidentiality.

Negative Consequences Maintaining Privacy and Confidentiality in a Clinical Setting

If privacy and confidentiality are not maintained it might put the patient under psychological distress and depression. While sharing information the nurse has to uphold patient confidentiality and privacy by adhering to all applicable laws and ethical standards. Failure to do so may harm the nurse-patient relationship and have legal repercussions for both the nurse and the employer they work for. In the workplace and off-duty in all settings, including social media or any other means of contact, the nurse has a responsibility to uphold the confidentiality of all patient information, both personal and clinical. Nurses should take all necessary precautions to protect data security whenever they use electronic communications or deal with electronic health records.

Points to be Remembered to Maintain Privacy and Confidentiality

- Build a trusting relationship with the patient and their family members.
- Take written informed consent from them whenever any data is to be used for academic or quality assurance activities.
- Have a quiet conversation with patients or coworkers whenever sensitive health information is the content of the conversation, e.g., breaking the bad news.
- Exception of disclosure should be only permitted if it is a threat to the patient's life or if there is a threat to public health and violation of existing legal requirements.
- Avoid sensitive or private conversations in public or semipublic areas of the ward.
- Strictly maintain access to computer recorded data through passwords to avoid authorized access. While using electronic media for sharing patient-related information, make sure both parties are using encryption technologies and make sure it is sent to the correct people only.
- Maintain the organizational policy for the maintenance of patient privacy.

HONESTY AND INTEGRITY: TRUTH-TELLING

Veracity or truth-telling is another vital component in a nurse-patient relationship. It is the moral duty of nurses, to be honest with their patients. It works on the principle of accuracy and truth-telling. Veracity means being truthful with patients, families, and colleagues. Nurses must be honest and tell truth, even if the truth may lead to distress or anxiety for the patient.

Integrity on the other hand in nursing denotes "acting according to the regulatory beliefs of the hospital or institution a nurse works for and upholding their standards and expectations regarding patient care." In clinical situations loss of integrity occurs in certain scenario such as providing false reassurance regarding patient care, prognosis, etc.

Importance of Veracity and Integrity In Nursing

The following are the reasons for the maintenance of veracity by nurses:

- Veracity demonstrates respect for patient's right of being treated equally and fairly.
- They promote the autonomy of decision-making of their patients.
- Honesty strengthens the interpersonal relationship between nurse and patient.
- It promotes honesty on the part of patients and also thus helps to make realistic health goals.
- Improves the functioning of the healthcare team within the organization as the professional relationship gets stronger.

Points to Remember for Maintaining Veracity and Integrity in Nursing

- Admitting mistakes and facing the consequences of mistakes for the sake of their patients. For example, admitting administration of a wrong dose/drug before it threatens the patient's life.
- Acknowledging and accepting the challenging health issues of patients that are interfering with the care initiatives.
- *Maintaining accurate health records*: Nurses must be honest in documenting their patient-related findings which help in the continuity of care across the health care team.

- *Accepting own limitations and asking for help*: Irrespective of their work experiences nurses must ask for help when it is not possible to manage alone.
- Regular quality assessment is to be done to maintain the standard of practice and identify any shortcomings at the earliest.
- Take informed consent from patients concerning their medical treatments or intervention. The patient must make knowledgeable decisions.
- Avoid giving false assurance. There are situations where nurses value the emotions of patients and their family members. But they should always know the truth about their patient. Disclosing information with utmost dignity and respect is the ultimate responsibility of the nurse.

Consequences of Lack of Veracity and Integrity in Nursing

Integrity in nursing is essential for building relationships with patients and delivering moral, high-quality care. Loss of integrity is acting dishonestly. The consequences due to lack of veracity and integrity in nursing has been depicted in **Figure 4.7**.

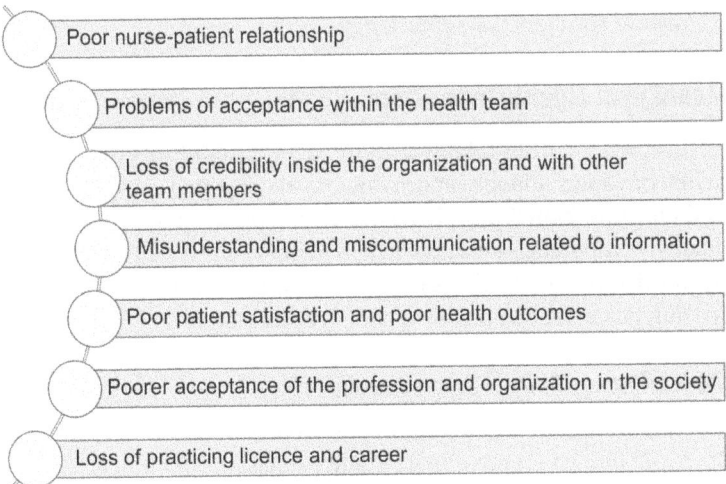

Fig. 4.7: Consequences of lack of veracity and integrity in nursing.

TRUST AND CREDIBILITY: FIDELITY AND LOYALTY

The nursing profession lies in the foundation of the quality of being faithful. "Faith" means trust and faithfulness implies trust. Trust, credibility, fidelity, and loyalty are interrelated concepts. A nurse needs to gain the loyalty of the patients, coworkers, and hospital administration. The loyalty can be demonstrated by talking to patients who require assistance and making an effort to allay their worries. Building trust increases a patient's likelihood of cooperating with treatments and aids nurses in better understanding the requirements of those under their care. Patients who have faith in their medical professionals are less stressed and may heal more quickly from injuries or illnesses.

Meaning of the Terms

- **Trust:** The confidence of believing that somebody is good, honest, sincere, and will not harm.
- **Credibility:** The quality that somebody has that makes people believe or trust him/her
- **Fidelity:** The Latin word "fides" means faithfulness. It is concerned with keeping promises, integrity, and honesty.
- **Loyalty:** Loyalty can be defined as the attachment that characterizes someone to be consistent in their feelings, affections, or habits toward someone, or something.

Meaning of Fidelity In Nursing

As discussed, earlier fidelity is defined as "faithfulness to a person, belief, or cause." Fidelity in nursing means nurses must remain true to their professional promises such as the promise to provide high-quality, competent, safe, and efficient patient care. It also means being supportive of patient decisions, promoting patient autonomy, and striving toward the improvement of the profession.

Nurse's Responsibility in Developing Fidelity
- Listen carefully to the patients, observe for nonverbal cues.
- Avoid being judgmental of patient's decisions or choices.
- Try to keep words given to patients.
- Keep calm even when patients are argumentative.

- Make a priority of the needs of the assigned patients.
- Promote patient autonomy by educating them and helping them to make the right choices.
- Always support the decision of patients and families.
- Being faithful to the nursing profession.
- Protect the confidentiality of patients.
- Fulfill the commitments toward patients and colleagues.

Effect of Fidelity in Nursing

High levels of trust in the healthcare setting is associated with many benefits such as:
- Perception of better care.
- Greater acceptance and adherence to the treatment, regular follow-up.
- Lower anxiety among patients and the health care team.
- Greater patient autonomy and shared decision-making.
- Create a conducive atmosphere for the development and maintenance of good practices.

Consequences of Lack of Fidelity In Nursing

The following are the consequences of lack of fidelity in nursing:
- Poor nurse-patient relationship due to lack of confidence.
- The increased cost of healthcare is due to mental distress.
- Decreased sense of dependability as a healthcare team member might disrupt the team's performance.
- Lack of adherence to institutional stand of practice affects the quality of service.
- Career disruption in the form of loss of job and loss of credibility with colleagues.
- Poor social acceptability of the nursing profession.

Fidelity in nursing refers to a nurse's commitment to upholding ethical commitments such as the promise to deliver excellent, knowledgeable, secure, and effective patient care. Additionally, it entails fostering patient autonomy, supporting patient decisions, and advancing the field. Nursing fidelity shows a nurse's commitment to providing skilled patient care in a just honest and responsible manner. Nursing fidelity entails exhibiting ideas of loyalty and faithfulness, the value of keeping promises, and teamwork in patient care.

ADVOCACY

Advocacy for patients, work environment, nursing education, and practice, and for advancing the profession.

The dictionary meaning of "advocate" is a person who supports and speaks in favor of somebody or some public plan/action. "Advocates" are mostly hired professional who supports their clients in terms of monitory benefit. Advocacy can be defined as an act of so-called "whistle blowing" that is, making known public, institutions or practices that are deemed unethical or negligent.

Nurses are the direct care provider to their clients in the clinical setting or the community setting. They act as the mediator between the patient and the entire health team. Advocacy is a regular practice in day-to-day nursing care. Patient care advocacy was valued by Florence Nightingale as we remember she advocated for the needs of soldiers of Crimean war. Since the movement of "patient advocacy" in 1970s nursing was viewed as the ideal profession to practice. Advocacy for nursing stems from a philosophy of nursing where it is believed that nursing practice is the support of an individual to promote his or her well-being, as understood by that individual.

The advocacy process comprises four steps:

- ❖ Assess the demands of the patients while taking into account their medical histories, philosophical beliefs, and level of consciousness.
- ❖ Identify the patient's objectives, including the types of treatments they want.
- ❖ Establish an advocacy strategy to achieve those objectives, which may entail collaborating with other members of their medical team.
- ❖ Evaluate the impact of their advocacy, taking into account the patient's, family's, and team's satisfaction.

Types of Advocacies

1. Case advocacy is directed toward changing the life of an individual. For example, patient care advocacy.
2. Class advocacy focuses on altering the system of opportunities itself to advance the interests of organizations, or communities rather than primarily on the client's opportunity choices. For instance, advocating for the workplace, nursing education and

practice, and the advancement of the profession.
- **Advocacy for the patients**, is the philosophical basis of nurses which supports an individual to promote his or her well-being. Thus advocacy for them not only involves preserving the rights of the human being but also maintaining **human dignity, promoting patient equality and providing freedom from suffering** allowing decisions about their health care choices.
- **Advocacy for work environment** making necessary changes through advocacy in the work environment to ensure safe work practice (e.g., adequate supply of personnel protective equipment during COVID pandemic, adequate nurse-patient ratio, unbiased appraisal for increment, etc.).
- **Advocacy for nursing education, practice, and advancing the profession** includes influencing decision-makers and legislators to make changes in the existing system of education and practice as per the need of the society (for example, introduction of nurse practitioner course in India). It also includes the creation of new courses, opportunities for continuing education/in-service education, and utilization of specialized nurses in specific units for better care of patients.

Measures to Enhance Advocacy for Patients

- ❖ **Educate patients:** Educate patients regarding their health and well-being, and their disease condition which must include the details of their disease and options of treatment modalities available. The knowledge should be imparted in simple terms as per the understanding level of the clients and community. Educating patients will improve their quality of life (e.g., improves acceptance of chronic conditions) and health-related expenses (such as preventing patients from unnecessary visits to hospitals) as they become capable of managing their acute or chronic condition in place of medical management.
- ❖ **Encourage verbal expression of feelings:** Nurses must encourage patients to verbal expression of feelings with any members of health care teams.
- ❖ **Ensure safety:** Ensure the patient's safety while receiving treatment in a hospital by communicating with others about the client's needs so that it can be arranged on a priority basis.

- ❖ **Protect patients' rights:** Safeguarding patient's rights by making them aware of their rights is one way of enhancing patient advocacy.
- ❖ **Avoiding medical errors:** Avoiding medical errors and correcting mistakes are the best ways to demonstrate patient advocacy.
- ❖ **Connect patients to resources:** Assisting patients in locating resources both inside and outside the hospital is one of the ways to promote patient advocacy.

Measures to Enhance Advocacy for Professional Issues

- ❖ Keep aware of the changes in the profession.
- ❖ Get informed regarding the standards of practice.
- ❖ Identify the priority-based emerging problem.
- ❖ Approach the administrators with relevant data.
- ❖ Stay respectful and humble during the negotiation.
- ❖ Take the help of local or national nurses organizations if necessary.

Benefits and Ill Effects of Advocacy

The positive benefits of advocacy for nurses involved are:
- ❖ Enhancement of nurse-patient relationship
- ❖ Helps the nurses to understand the patient's need
- ❖ Improves patient outcomes.
- ❖ Professional autonomy and efficiency in decision making
- ❖ Enhanced participation of nurses in policymaking
- ❖ Improvement of the public image and professional status of nurses.
- ❖ The various negative consequences of nursing advocacy are frustration and anger, lowering of status such as a demotion in the institutional hierarchy, and being labeled by peers as an instigator, troublemakers, or whistle-blower.

■ CHAPTER HIGHLIGHTS

- ❖ In nursing education, it is becoming more important to promote professional values due to the complexity and increasing number of ethical dilemmas in care settings.
- ❖ Socialization refers to the process by which individuals gain the knowledge, skills, and attitudes that are necessary for them to be able to contribute to their community.

- ❖ Human dignity, integrity, compassion, and fairness are significant professional nursing principles that provide a foundation for standards, professional practice, and evaluation.
- ❖ In the nursing profession, the concept of human dignity is basic, nebulous, multifaceted, and multidimensional.
- ❖ Nurses must develop and use skills in critical thinking, effective communication, teamwork, and evidence-based clinical knowledge to assure the quality of patient care and safety under the new healthcare delivery paradigm.

MULTIPLE CHOICE QUESTIONS

1. Which of the following is an example of professional values relevant to nursing?
   - a. Human dignity
   - b. Power
   - c. Hedonism
   - d. Achievement
2. Which of the following is considered the central, dominant, and unifying focus of nursing?
   - a. Advocacy
   - b. Privacy
   - c. Caring
   - d. Honesty
3. The verbal and nonverbal expression of sorrow or concern is called as
   - a. Empathy
   - b. Sympathy
   - c. Conscientiousness
   - d. Compassion
4. The selfless concern for the well-being of the others is?
   - a. Altruism
   - b. Empathy
   - c. Sympathy
   - d. Advocacy
5. Truth-telling is also called as:
   - a. Fidelity
   - b. Veracity
   - c. Hedonism
   - d. Benevolence

ANSWERS

| 1. a | 2. c | 3. b | 4. a | 5. a |

BIBLIOGRAPHY

1. Abbasinia M, Ahmadi F, Kazemnejad A. Patient advocacy in nursing: A concept analysis. Nurs Ethics. 2020;27(1):141-51.
2. Andersson EK, Willman A, Sjöström-Strand A, Borglin G. Registered nurses' descriptions of caring: a phenomenographic interview study. BMC Nurs. 2015;14:16.
3. Baillie L, Black S. Professional Values in Nursing, 1st edition. London: Routledge; 2014.

4. Breeding J, Turner de S. Registered nurses' lived experience of advocacy within a critical care unit: a phenomenological study. Aust Crit Care. 2002;15(3):110-7.
5. Burnard P, Chapman CM, Smallman S. Professional and ethical issues in nursing. 3rd edition. Edinburgh: Baillière Tindall; 2004.
6. Hadadian-Chaghaei F, Haghani F, Taleghani F, Feizi A, Alimohammadi N. Nurses as gifted artists in caring: an analysis of nursing care concept. Iran J Nurs Midwifery Res. 2022;27(2):125-33.
7. Hanks RG. The lived experience of nursing advocacy. Nurs Ethics. 2008;15(4):468-77.
8. Kalaitzidis E, Jewell P. The Concept of Advocacy in Nursing: A Critical Analysis. Health Care Manag (Frederick). 2020;39(2):77-84.
9. Lee JJ, Yang SC. Professional socialisation of nursing students in a collectivist culture: a qualitative study. BMC Med Educ. 2019;19(1):254.
10. Osteen PJ. Motivations, values, and conflict resolution: students' integration of personal and professional identities. J Soc Work Educ. 2011; 47(3): 423–44.
11. Pai HC, Hui HC, Huang Y. Factors that Influence Professional Socialization in Nursing Students: A Multigroup Analysis. Open J Nurs., 2021; 11(3), 104-20.
12. Poorchangizi B, Borhani F, Abbaszadeh A, Mirzaee M, Farokhzadian J. Professional values of nurses and nursing students: a comparative study. BMC Med Educ. 2019;19(1):438.
13. Sadeghi Avval Shahr H, Yazdani S, Afshar L. Professional socialization: an analytical definition. J Med Ethics Hist Med. 2019;12:17.
14. Sagiv L, Roccas S, Cieciuch J, Schwartz SH. Personal values in human life. Nat Hum Behav. 2017;1(9):630-9.
15. Salisu WJ, Dehghan Nayeri N, Yakubu I, Ebrahimpour F. Challenges and facilitators of professional socialization: A systematic review. Nurs Open. 2019;6(4):1289-98.
16. Schmidt BJ, McArthur EC. Professional nursing values: A concept analysis. Nurs Forum. 2018;53(1):69-75.
17. Smith A. An analysis of altruism: a concept of caring. J Adv Nurs. 1995;22(4):785-90.
18. Swardt H C, Rensburg GH, Oosthuizen M. Supporting students in professional socialisation: Guidelines for professional nurses and educators. Int J Africa Nurs Sci. 2017; 6(6): 1–7.
19. Turale S, Kunaviktikul W. The contribution of nurses to health policy and advocacy requires leaders to provide training and mentorship. Int Nurs Rev. 2019;66(3):302-304.
20. Uustal DB. Values clarification in nursing: application to practice. Am J Nurs. 1978;78(12):2058-63.
21. Zarshenas L, Sharif F, Molazem Z, Khayyer M, Zare N, Ebadi A. Professional socialization in nursing: A qualitative content analysis. Iran J Nurs Midwifery Res. 2014;19(4):432-8.

UNIT 3

Ethics and Bioethics

CHAPTER 5

Ethics and Bioethics

Shiv Kumar Mudgal, Rakhi Gaur

Learning Objectives

Upon completion of this chapter, the readers should be able to:
- Differentiate between ethics and morality.
- Define the key terms used in ethics and bioethics.
- Understand the ethical theories and ethical principles.
- Apply ethical principles in nursing practice.

■ MEANING OF ETHICS, MORALITY, BIOETHICS

Ethics

The word ethics is derived from the ancient Greek word "ethikos", which means "relating to one's character". "Ethikos" derives its name from the root word of "ethos". It refers to customs, habitual usages, and conduct. It is about defining the moral dimension in life including duties, responsibilities, justice, conscience, and other social concerns. It is the discipline of philosophy that investigates the concept of right and wrong. Ethics is concerned with the study of moral behavior. The study of ethics is the study of one's logically defined responsibilities, obligations, and commitments. Ethics is profoundly grounded in the legal system and reflects our society's political beliefs.

Some of the definitions of ethics are given below:
- Rushworth Kidder defines ethics as —*"the science of the ideal human character* or *the science of moral duty"*
- Richard William Paul and Linda Elder define ethics as "a set of concepts and principles that guide us in determining what behavior helps or harms sentient creatures."
- Ethics is the open, rational, and public assessment of alternative actions relative to theories and rules.

Morality

Sometimes the term "moral" is misunderstood when it is meant to mean "ethics." Morality is usually a personal, private standard of conduct, character, or attitude. An active conscience, awareness of guilt, shame, and hope can often be the first sign of the morality of a situation. Moral behavior is defined as conforming to practice or culture. It frequently reflects a person's religious or personal convictions, as well as his or her wish to protect the freedom to die.

Bioethics

Bioethics is the science that deals with the rightness and wrongness of actions within the scope of medicine, nursing, and allied health. It is the study of ethics concerning health and human life (e.g., decisions about abortion or end of life). Bioethics is the application of general ethical principles to healthcare. Bioethics can be described as a subcategory within ethics. It addresses ethical issues such as those that arise from technological advancements and advances in science. Stem cells, cloning, and genetic engineering are some of the most important bioethical issues.

An *ethical theory* is a moral principle or a set of moral principles that can be used in assessing what is morally right or morally wrong. The major ethical theories which help to provide guidelines for ethical decision-making are enlisted in **Table 5.1**.

Table 5.1: Ethical theories.

Virtue ethics (Proponent—Aristotle)
- Virtues are excellences of intellect or character that are developed throughout one's life through personal efforts, training, and practice.
- All human beings have an inborn nature or virtues to decide "what is good or bad" which helps them to choose the right course of action during the ethical dilemma

Utilitarianism
- This theory holds the "principle of greatest happiness" which postulates that any action which promotes happiness is considered as good.
- If the results or the consequences of the action do not produce happiness, it is considered wrong.

Kantianism (Proponent—Immanuel Kant)
- This theory is also called "deontology" which means "duty" or "obligation".
- This theory affirms the importance of following moral law, rules, and principles.
- Kantianism asserts that the rightness or wrongness of actions is decided if it is performed based on some set of rules or sense of duty than the consequence of actions.

ETHICAL PRINCIPLES

The principles of biomedical ethics include four principles that serve as guidelines for fundamental moral behaviors. These include autonomy, nonmaleficence, beneficence, and justice. These are the universal norms shared by all persons committed to morality that help in choosing the best action during complex situations of ethical dilemmas. The meanings of the fundamental principles of ethics are described **Table 5.2**.

Table 5.2: Fundamental ethical principles.

Principle	Meaning
Beneficence	This principle emphasizes the importance of *"do good"* or acting for the benefit of the patient.
Nonmaleficence	This principle emphasizes the importance of *"do no harm"* or prevent harm.
Autonomy	This principle emphasizes the right to determine for own treatment or choices of actions (self-determination).
Justice	This principle emphasizes the fairness or equitableness and appropriate distribution of health care resources and services.

APPLICATION OF ETHICAL PRINCIPLES

Ethical principles are guiding or governing principles. These principles are generally accepted by the public and are founded on humane aspects. Ethical decisions reflect the best interests of both the client and society. By adopting ethical concepts, nurses can become more organized in their ethical problem-solving. These principles can help nurses analyze conflicts and can also be utilized as a framework for resolving ethical issues. Autonomy, beneficence, nonmaleficence, veracity, integrity, justice, accountability, the standard of the best care, and obligations are some of the ethical principles explored in this chapter **(Table 5.3)**.

❖ **Autonomy:** This is an ancient concept (derived from the ancient Greek words "autos," meaning "self," and "nomos," meaning "rule") that refers to a patient's right to self-determination, independence, and the ability to make their own choices. It outlines the individual's freedom to make their decisions and the ability to follow through on those choices, even if they are not supported by the health care provider. When autonomy is maintained, each person's individuality is respected. This principle is respected by

Table 5.3: Summary of ethical principles applied in nursing practice.

Ethical principles	Application in practice
Autonomy	Allow patients to make decisions without coercion or judgment
Beneficence	Doing the right thing for patients
Nonmaleficence	No intentional or unintentional harm
Veracity	Being truthful with patients
Fidelity	Being loyal and true to their professional duties through efficiently rendering high-quality and safe care
Justice	A group of patients must receive equal and fair care
Accountability	All professional and personal consequences for nursing actions must be accepted
Standard of the best interest	When a client is unable to make an informed decision regarding their health care, a decision is made on their behalf
Obligations	Rights that are owed to others

nurses who recognize each client's uniqueness and have the right to decide their own goals. Respecting autonomy implies that the nurse will regard the client's right to make an informed decision, even if they are not in the best interests of the client. Autonomy, as an ethical principle, is founded on the belief that every individual is capable of choosing their actions. The client's decision-making capacity decides whether they have the freedom to select. This also entails showing respect to others.

Clients' rights to make their own decisions are the foundation of informed consent. However, autonomy can be limited under certain circumstances in which client-initiated actions cause a delay in the recovery or treatment. For example, avoidance of using precautions after the diagnosis of a sexually transmitted disease (STDs). In the case of contagious disease (e.g., COVID-19), the law and healthcare systems can force the client to have the necessary precautions to safeguarding others. To stop the infection from spreading, it is necessary to force an individual into isolation.

Chapter 5: Ethics and Bioethics

■ **Critical Thinking**
A 26-year-old female was involved in an accident. Her head struck the front windshield of her car, causing blunt force trauma. She did not lose consciousness and had no neurological impairment symptoms. Nonetheless, she has a significant head wound that is constantly bleeding. The lady resisted treatment, asserting that she felt well and refusing to have her head wound sutured. She desires to leave the hospital. Although a computed tomography (CT) scan and sutures would be in the best interest of the patient, the patient is an adult with full mental capacity. Does the nurse accept the client's choice to leave the treatment hospital?

- ❖ **Beneficence** is "doing right." It is an absolute necessity for all healthcare providers. This principle considers that the primary goal is to be able to provide quality care for the clients who seek it. Beneficence refers to the ethical principle of the duty to promote good and prevent harm. Nurses must have the obligation to do well. This means taking steps that are beneficial to clients and their caregivers. The definition of good goes beyond providing competent care to the clients. A holistic approach to client care is essential. This encompasses the client's thoughts and emotions, as well as their family members and other's significant desires and requirements.
  Two elements of beneficence are providing benefits and balancing harms. This principle requires that health care workers not only avoid harm but also benefit patients and promote their welfare. Therefore, the nurse is obligated to behave in the best interests of the patient under the beneficence principle. Providing suitable positions with comfort devices for a client experiencing respiratory distress is an act of beneficence. However, doing good might equally increase the likelihood of causing harm. For example, a nurse has started a blood transfusion to save the patient's life but the patient might start having some mild allergic reactions. Sometimes, implementing the principle of beneficence can be difficult because it is hard to determine what is best for someone else and who is most qualified to make that decision.
- ❖ **Nonmaleficence** refers to the obligation to "do no harm." As a core obligation, health care professionals must practice nonmaleficence. Both the Hippocratic Oath and the Nightingale Pledge declare that healthcare professionals should not do harm to patients. Nonmaleficence encourages nurses to consider the

benefits and risks of treatment with great care. This principle asserts the ethical question: "Will this treatment modality cause greater harm or more good for the client?" A possible factor to be considered while answering the above-said question is that the treatment should offer reasonable benefits and it should not be expensive, painful, or inconvenient.

It is a legal necessity that healthcare professionals do not injure their patients, whether intentionally or unintentionally. However, the principle of nonmaleficence in health care is often broken to achieve a greater benefit for the client in the long term. For example, a client might have to undergo painful surgeries and chemotherapy to remove cancerous growths. This could prolong his life. It is also worth noting that unintentional harm in nursing is relatively acceptable. For instance, a nurse may grasp a client who has fallen to the ground, resulting in bruises on the client's arm. In addition, the principle of nonmaleficence necessitates that nurses must safeguard vulnerable populations such as children, the mentally ill, the unconscious, and someone unable to defend themselves. Preventing drug interactions and raising the bedside rails to prevent falls are some of the nursing actions under this principle.

- ❖ **Veracity** is truthfulness. It means that the healthcare provider must tell the truth, not deceive clients or intentionally mislead them. The principle of veracity, although not a legal requirement, is a foundation for a trusting relationship between a client and nurse, which is essential to any therapeutic relationship. Nurses are sometimes hesitant to convey the bad news of their condition because they are uncomfortable doing so. However, feeling uneasy is not a good enough excuse to keep clients from learning the truth about their diagnosis, treatments, or prognosis. While nurses have an obligation to be truthful, clients have the right to access information about their condition. *Placebo medication* use is a common example of veracity being violated. Medical errors are another issue that has been related to this principle. Many believe that medical errors should not be disclosed if clients aren't hurt. However, reporting errors has an essential duty of the nurse to prevent further associated consequences. Although it may seem easy to disclose the truth, it can be difficult to determine how much truth to share. This may look simple, but in practice, the choices are not always easy.

Chapter 5: Ethics and Bioethics

■ **Critical Thinking**
Is it acceptable for a nurse to disclose the truth if doing so may cause harm?
Is it justifiable for a nurse to tell a lie if the lie will relieve anxiety or fear?
It is reasonable for a nurse to lie to dying or sick people?

❖ **Fidelity:** The ethical foundation for nurse-client relationships is the concept of fidelity. It describes faithfulness to agreements and keeping promises. An individual is obligated to keep all promises made to him/her and others. Clients have the right to expect nurses and other health care professionals to act in their best interest. In the field of health care, fidelity refers to a professional's commitment to the promises and duties that come with their profession. Fidelity is the foundation of accountability and it upholds client advocacy. Nurses can demonstrate fidelity by communicating the client's point of view with other health team members and by supporting the patient's decision, even if the nurse does not even agree with his or her preferences.

■ **Critical Thinking**
A patient requested not to disclose his terminal diagnosis to his family members. He further states that they would likely disregard his wishes and there is a chance of rejection from the family members in anticipation of his terminal stage of illness. How can the nurse acknowledge the need to protect the patient's privacy and support his family?

❖ **Justice:** The principle of justice rests on fairness. It is the obligation to be fair to all. It states that everyone has the right to equitable treatment regardless of color, gender, or marital status. The American Nurses Association (ANA) Code of Ethics for Nurses (2014) begins with the concept of justice: "The nurse in all professional relations practices compassion and respect for each individual's inherent dignity, worth, and uniqueness, without regard to social or economic status, personal attributes or the nature of their health problems." The ethical principle of justice mandates that nursing care should be distributed equally, based on need, and priority basis. There are many situations in which nurses must act with justice. For example, a nurse visiting a client at home finds her feeling depressed. She knows that she can help the client by spending some extra time talking to her. However, this would be a time-consuming task for her next client who requires palliative nursing care. Therefore, to promote justice, the nurse has to weigh the significant benefits and burdens of both the clients and act accordingly. According to the American Nurses Association (ANA; 1991), there are three sorts of conduct that are deemed unjust: (i) When implementing policies/rules, there is discrimination and arbitrary uneven treatment, (ii) taking undue advantage of another, and (iii) making false or derogatory comments about someone else.

■ Critical Thinking
Two patients are admitted for kidney transplantation.
❖ A 70-year-old patient with diabetes and prostate cancer.
❖ A 35-year-old male with polycystic kidney disease.
How would the nurse protect the patient's right to equality or fairness in availing treatment?

❖ **Accountability:** Accountability is a fundamental part of professional nursing practice. It is often called the "hallmark" of professionalism. Professional accountability and responsibility are essential for nurses. According to the Code of Ethics for Nurses, accountability is defined as being "responsible to oneself and others for one's conduct," whereas responsibility is defined as "the specific obligations for the fulfillment of a particular role." The ethical nurse can articulate the rationale behind each action and is aware of the standards for which they will be held accountable. Nurses who are held accountable for their actions commit themselves. This allows them to learn from both successes and failures. Professional practice requires accountability. Nurses can make judgments in many situations and all aspects of nursing practice can be considered accountable, including assuring/ providing quality of care, the delegation of work, following policies and procedures, following the guidelines set by the organization, ensuring confidentiality, and patient advocacy and proficiency in the clinical skills. Nursing professionals use their knowledge, skills, and judgment to make evidence-based decisions that are in the best interests of the patient. Accountability is a consequence of autonomy. For example, if a physician prescribed a drug incorrectly, the nurse is also accountable for administering it. Nurse practitioner has autonomy to assess, diagnose and preserve treatment to patients as a result she/he is accountable for these independent practices.

- ❖ **Standard for best interest:** The standard of best interests was created to assist in surrogate decision-making. It was first used by courts to make end-of-life decisions about incompetent clients. This refers to a decision made on the patient's health care while the client is unable to do so. The principles of beneficence, nonmaleficence, and beneficence should guide the determination of the best interest. After examining all relevant information, the standard of best interest demands that a good faith determination be made about which treatment(s) or actions would result in a better outcome for the client. This decision must be made in compliance with medical and ethical standards. Paternalism occurs when healthcare providers make unilateral decisions that are not in the best interests of the patient. This is because clients who are unable to make their own decisions can be rendered incapable by the providers. Paternalism is not usually considered ethical but can be justifiable in certain circumstances such as the condition in which incompetency limits a patient's choices.
- ❖ **Obligations:** Obligations are the duty of an individual, a profession to fulfill and respect the rights of others. Legal and moral obligations are the two sorts of obligations in the context of health care services **(Fig. 5.1)**.

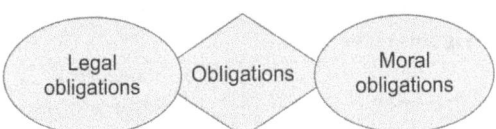

Fig. 5.1: Types of obligations.

1. **Legal obligations:** Legal duties are those that have been formalized into statutes and are enforceable in court. Nurses, for example, are required by law to provide clients with safe and appropriate care.
2. **Moral obligations:** These are obligations that are not enforced by the law but are based on moral and ethical principles. As an example, a nurse who is providing first aid measures to the victim of an automobile accident adheres to her moral obligation.

Every day, nurses are faced with many obligations in which they must make decisions based on what is right and what is wrong. However, safeguarding the rights of the clients often contradicts professional responsibilities and institutional arrangements. Therefore, these two perspectives must be balanced so that quality care can be delivered.

CHAPTER HIGHLIGHTS

- Nursing ethics is concerned with ethical dilemmas that occur in the practice of nursing as well as ethical decisions made by nurses.
- Morality refers only to your private standards of behavior, character, and attitude.
- There are majorly three types of ethical theories: Virtue ethics, utilitarianism, and Kantianism
- Nurses are responsible for their own decisions and for supporting clients who make moral decisions or for whom others make decisions.
- Ethical decisions must be based on principles such as autonomy and beneficence, nonmaleficence, and veracity. Justice, accountability, the standard for best care, and obligations.

MULTIPLE CHOICE QUESTIONS

1. The word ethos means:
   a. Conduct
   b. Habit
   c. Characters
   d. Hobbies
2. The immunization of a child may be uncomfortable to administer, but the advantages of illness prevention, for both the patient and society as a whole, outweigh the short-term discomforts. Which principle is applicable in this case?
   a. Fidelity
   b. Beneficence
   c. Nonmaleficence
   d. Respect for autonomy
3. If unable to make judgments, a person may choose to decide certain medical treatments, which are listed in a document called the:
   a. Advance directives
   b. Living will
   c. Informed consent
   d. Durable power of attorney
4. The science that deals with the rightness and wrongness of actions is called as
   a. Ethics
   b. Epistemology
   c. Axiology
   d. Metaphysics
5. Which of the following is an example of ethical theory?
   a. Beneficence
   b. Deontology
   c. Justice
   d. Veracity

ANSWERS

| 1. a | 2. b | 3. a | 4. a | 5. b |

BIBLIOGRAPHY

1. Alhazmi F. The Ethical Challenge of Conflicts of Interest in Healthcare. Retrieved from https://dsc.duq.edu/etd/1780.
2. Flite CA, Harman LB. Code of ethics: principles for ethical leadership. Perspect Health Inf Manag. 2013;10(Winter):1d. Epub 2013 Jan 1. PMID: 23346028
3. Haddad LM, Geiger RA. Nursing Ethical Considerations. [Updated 2021 Aug 30]. In: StatPearls [Internet]. Treasure Island (FL): StatPearls Publishing; 2022 Jan-. Available from: https://www.ncbi.nlm.nih.gov/books/NBK526054/
4. Jahn WT. The 4 basic ethical principles that apply to forensic activities are respect for autonomy, beneficence, nonmaleficence, and justice. Journal of chiropractic medicine. 2011 Sep;10(3):225.
5. Parandeh A, Khaghanizade M, Mohammadi E, Mokhtari-Nouri J. Nurses' human dignity in education and practice: An integrated literature review. Iran J Nurs Midwifery Res. 2016 Jan-Feb;21(1):1-8.
6. Shahriari M, Mohammadi E, Abbaszadeh A, Bahrami M. Nursing ethical values and definitions: A literature review. Iran J Nurs Midwifery Res. 2013 Jan;18(1):1-8.
7. Stark L, Hedgecoe A. A practical guide to research ethics. The Sage Handbook of Qualitative Methods in Health Research. New York: Sage. 2010.
8. Varkey B. Principles of Clinical Ethics and Their Application to Practice. Med Princ Pract. 2021;30(1):17-28.

CHAPTER 6

Ethical Issues and Ethical Dilemma

Rakhi Gaur, Shiv Kumar Mudgal

Learning Objectives

Upon completion of this chapter, the readers should be able to:
* Understand about different ethical issues encountered during clinical practice.
* Discuss ethical and legal issues related to beginning of life.
* Describe ethical and legal issues encountered at the end-of-life.
* Explain ethical and legal issues faced during psychiatric care.
* Practice use of ethical principles and solving ethical dilemmas.

■ MEANING OF ETHICAL DILEMMA

Ethical and legal considerations are inherent to the profession of nursing and nurses routinely face ethical dilemmas in their daily care practices. As a nurse, it is important to establish and nurture relationships with patients and their families. Ethically and legally, nurses are accountable for the actions they take and those they delegate care. All nurses must adhere to professional codes and standards of practice in nursing. The role of nurse managers and leaders is to ensure that nurses are competent and able to provide safe and ethical nursing care while adhering to all applicable laws and regulations. Ethical and legal difficulties frequently become enmeshed in the modern healthcare system.

What Does Ethical Dilemma Mean?

An ethical dilemma is a contradiction between two or more ethical standards. When two or more of the ethical principles are at odds, there is an ethical dilemma. There is no right or wrong choice. The circumstances will determine which option is the best. A nurse must decide between two equally unsatisfactory options when confronted with an ethical dilemma. Ethical analysis can be a complex science. Even when a problem seems resolved, sometimes there are still questions. This creates an emotional pain for both the person and the nurse.

The truth is that ethical issues are often not easy to resolve. A dilemma in ethics is when there are multiple morally acceptable actions that cannot be followed. There are two types of ethical dilemmas in these situations—(1) ethical conflict and (2) ethical behavior. One of the most common ethical dilemmas faced in critical care is to go for treatment or allocate critical care resource. But how does a health worker know if this is an ethical dilemma? Before any decision model can apply, it must first be established if the true ethical dilemma exists. There are three criteria that can be used to determine whether a clinical situation is morally or ethically problematic:

1. An awareness of the different options.
2. A problem that offers options.
3. More than two options, each with true or "good", aspects. The choice of one option may compromise the other.

Nurses frequently find themselves in an unpleasant situation regarding what to do and what not to do. For example, what should a nurse say to a patient with pancreatic carcinoma? This difficulty occurs when the ideals of honesty and nonmaleficence contradict. It also contradicts the autonomy principle. The client's right to make an informed decision is violated if they are not informed.

Before taking any action, it is important to pause, raise awareness in a group, validate assumptions, identify patterns of thought or behavior, and encourage reflection and inquiry. Some of the ethical dilemmas which are being discussed in this chapter are conflict of interest, paternalism, deception, confidentiality and privacy, informed consent and refusal, allocation of scare health resources, new technologies and whistle-blowing, etc.

■ CONFLICT OF INTEREST

Definition

- ❖ The College of Registered Nurses of British Columbia (CRNBC) mentions that "A conflict of interest occurs when a nurse's personal, business, commercial, political, academic or financial interests, or the nurse's family or friends, interfere with the nurse's professional responsibilities or a client's best interests."

Ethical Dilemma in Conflict of Interest

Conflicts of interests are a common problem in all areas of society. Unfortunately, this is also true for healthcare. Conflicts of interests arise when the nurses' primary goal of protecting the patient's interest is conflicted with their secondary goals. These conflicts are usually, but not always, related to financial gain. It is important for health care professionals to consider the consequences of their actions and weigh them against each other in order to neglect conflicts of interest. Avoid conflict of interest by choosing medical practices that have benefits greater than the risks.

Nursing and other healthcare professions have one goal—to contribute towards health promotion, illness prevention, health restoration, rehabilitation and a peaceful death of people. In order to achieve this goal, healthcare professionals must improve their skills and knowledge so that they can provide care for their patients and return them to their normal lives. It can be costly to achieve this goal. The conflict of interest created by managed care, as well as the competition for resources, is not to be ignored. Nurses may face workplace conflict as a result of competing loyalties, such as demands from patients' families, physicians, coworkers, healthcare organizations, and health insurance.

■ PATERNALISM

This principle is similar to beneficence, in that one person assumes authority to make decisions for another. Paternalism restricts freedom of choice. Most ethical theorists believe paternalism can only be justified to protect someone from harm.

It is "intentional overriding one person's actions or preferences by another person" (Beauchamp and Childress 2009). Many nurses justify paternalism by citing nonmaleficence and beneficence. A nurse may think that she or he knows best what the patient wants and will act accordingly based on their education and experience. This can interfere with the autonomy and right to self-determination of the patient. Nurses must be able to differentiate between paternalism and patient's choice of control. Additionally, they must help the patients to make informed decisions or respect their autonomy. It is paternalistic for a nurse not to inform a patient that his or her fever has risen or that he or she is experiencing irregular heartbeats. Hence, paternalism can be the decision of the nurse to disclose the information or not.

▪ DECEPTION

Deception is the act of causing someone to accept as true or valid what is false or invalid.

Definitions

- ❖ Dishonest or illegal methods that are used to get something, or to make people believe that something is true when it is not.
—Cambridge dictionary
- ❖ Deception is the act of deceiving someone or the state of being deceived by someone.
—Collins English dictionary

The codes of ethics and conduct for healthcare professionals address honesty and trust with respect to patient encounters. However, truth-telling (or being honest) versus deception (or being dishonest) have been identified in hospitals as an ethical problem, especially regarding diagnosis and prognosis disclosures. Dossa (2010) also states that deception may be an act or dishonesty, but can also be without lying. Deception can be described as not providing any information, withholding information or selecting the information that is most relevant, and choosing what information to share and not disclose. Critical care, palliative, and mental health are the most common areas in clinical practice where deception and truth-telling can become ethical dilemmas. There are also areas that could raise ethical concerns such as in placebo therapy, disclosures of human immune deficiency virus, and informed consent.

Truth-telling can also be described as the act of exchanging notions among moral agents (patients, relatives, and nurses) and their set of values and norms. These are derived from culture and personal religious beliefs and traditions. The issue of truth-telling can be approached differently in different settings and in different countries, cultures, and religions.

Ethical Dilemmas in Truth Telling

It is possible that patient care is dominated by nondisclosure. It is a part of the professional responsibility of nurses to "titrate" how much information they provide to patients. While this can be justified empirically since patients may be distressed if they are given too much information, deception is another matter. It is difficult to justify deception and it is rarely recognized in public. Sometimes, it is argued that some situations should not be called deception because the whole truth about a patient cannot be known and communicated. Therefore, one cannot know if the information they give is correct or incorrect. Sometimes deception is used to promote better care for patients such as reassurance (such as maintaining hope for the future), and sometimes due to organizational needs (such time considerations or concerns that a patient might become difficult to manage). Sometimes, nurses would use deception on the appeal of patient's families or because of consultant medical staff. Sometimes it is difficult to maintain deception while patients are aware of the severity of their physical condition. Most nurses justified their actions with the excuse of nonmaleficence. To keep patient's anxiety at bay about their condition, treatment or family, they used deceit. They believed they were helping their patients in a positive way by providing false information that would alleviate their anxiety.

■ CONFIDENTIALITY AND PRIVACY

The client's privacy is the responsibility of nurses. The confidential information must be disclosed only with the client's consent. Before exposing confidential information about a client or searching their personal belongings, nurses must obtain the client's permission. Ensuring confidentiality and privacy is vital to the practice of nursing. According to the American Nurses Association Code for Nurses (1985), upholding the integrity of the nursing profession requires strict adherence to the principles of privacy and confidentiality. Nursing care should be administered with a caring attitude that respects the client's privacy by closing the client's room door, knocking before entering, closing the bed's curtains before exposing the client, and

correctly draping the client for procedures. The idea of privacy, according to Badzek and Gross (1999), comprises the right to:
- Allow yourself to be alone (i.e., freedom from intrusion)
- Examine the integrity of the body (to consent to or refuse treatment) and
- Keep control over the sharing of personal data.

Privacy is a principle that a person has the right to restrict access to personal information. Privacy is not just an ethical value, but it is also a legal entitlement that is guaranteed by the legislation. Patients place their faith in nurses and share personal information with them. Respecting patient's privacy is a key responsibility for nurses. They are only permitted to share patient information with other healthcare personnel if absolutely required. Nurse leaders and managers must protect their employee's privacy by keeping religious beliefs and lifestyle choices private.

Patients are required to reveal personal information with nurses and healthcare providers. The principle of confidentiality is the protection of patient's private information from being disclosed to other members of the health care team. A nurse can only use personal information that a patient has shared with them. All information about patients must be kept secret by nurses. All nurses have a duty of confidentiality in regards to patient information. Confidentiality (respecting privileged information) is a core ethical principle and a basis of both medical and nursing ethics. It is the need to observe other's privacy and to keep specific information in tight confidence.

Access to electronic data is also a constantly growing concern that compromises privacy and confidentiality. The development of cellular phones, facsimile machines, and digital medical records has the potential to compromise information privacy. "Nurses at all levels have a duty to maintain confidentiality of all patient information, both personal and clinical, in the work setting and off duty in all venues including social media or any other means of communication" (ANA, 2015).

■ **Critical Thinking**
What are the circumstances in which breach of confidentiality is acceptable in the medical profession?

■ INFORMED CONSENT AND REFUSAL

The right to autonomy of the client is guaranteed by rules governing informed consent. If the client has all of the information necessary to make informed decisions about whether they consent to or refuse a treatment plan, they can do so. Clients and their representatives must be provided with sufficient information about the various treatment options so that consent can be made in an informed manner. Consent is the voluntary agreement to allow another person to perform a specific action. The client gives informed consent when he or she comprehends the intervention's purpose, risks, and benefits. In addition, they consent to the treatment by signing consent documents. Consent documents are especially required for any invasive procedures (accessing body tissues, organs, or cavities using an instrument). Clients must be legally competent in order to consent to medical operations. The legal obligation to acquire informed permission rests with the health care provider performing the treatment. Informed consent refers to a process that includes information and consent, rather than just signing a form (Switzer 1995). To obtain informed consent, the health care provider must instruct the client. The client cannot be forced to sign the consent by the provider of health care. The client is free to refuse information, waive informed consent and receive treatment. This decision must be recorded in his medical record. As long as the institutional policy allows, an informed consent may be waived in order to receive urgent medical or surgical intervention. A minor should have parental consent or guardian consent before any treatment is initiated. However, there are exceptions—in an emergency, where the minor's permission is required such as for the treatment of a sexually transmitted illness and when a court order or other legal authorization has been acquired. If the client is a juvenile and the guardian or parents refuse life-saving care, the court may overturn the decision.

For inappropriate disclosures of information, nurses could be held accountable. Here are some general guidelines to keep in mind:

❖ The responsibility to obtain informed consents primarily rest on the treating physician. However, a nurse might be found liable for a battery case (a legal proceeding) if she understands the patient has refused to be informed.

❖ The nurse can witness the client signing a consent form. In such situations, they may also have to make sure that the form

is in the chart. Client's signature must be witnessed by the registered nurse.
* If the nurse notices situations that render a signed consent form incorrect (for example, a change in the client's status), she should notify the physician. The nurse can refuse to perform a procedure until they have satisfied the informed consent requirements.

Ethical Liabilities While Obtaining Informed Consent

Informed consent refers to the client's voluntary consent to perform a procedure on him. Many court cases stem from clients claiming that they did not give informed consent prior to undergoing surgery or other invasive procedures. These legal proceedings are often against hospitals and doctors, but nurses may also be involved if they fail to provide enough information. The individual conducting the procedure is responsible for obtaining informed consent. A client can only give informed consent after receiving sufficient information about the treatment proposed, material risk involved (potential complications), other acceptable treatments, the hoped outcome for and the consequences of not receiving treatment. This information should be provided primarily by the physician. While nurses can supplement and reinforce the information provided by the physician, they should not be the only or primary source of informed consent information.

Some exceptional conditions, in which informed consent is not obligatory, include:
* In emergency situations, the client may not be able to consent because they are incapacitated or unconscious.
* Situations where the health care provider considers it medically unwise to disclose the risks and hazards. These situations could lead to illness, severe emotional distress, psychological damage, or the inability of the client to receive lifesaving treatments.

Role of Nurse in Obtaining Informed Consent

While nurses are not required to obtain informed consent for all nursing procedures, it is the duty of the nurse to explain to the client what is expected from his side. Informed consent is both legally and ethically required. It is an ethical notion that permits people to choose whether or not to get health care on their own. A legal process in which a patient or a legal representative grants authorization to undergo a procedure or treatment is known as *informed consent*. The three components of informed consent are knowledge, competency, and will. The patient must have full information and the patient must give fully competent to give their consent with a free willingness for undergoing the procedure. In order to give informed consent, the patient must be informed in such a way that he or she understands the choices as well as the risks and benefits of each option. This knowledge enables the patient to make well-informed choices. A summary of role of nurses in obtaining written informed consent is presented in **Box 6.1**.

■ **Critical Thinking**
What are the treatment procedures in the health care system in which informed consent is considered as mandatory?
What is the alternate action, if the client does not have the competency to provide informed consent?

Box 6.1: Nurse's role while obtaining written consent are described here.
- Verifying that the patient was given all the information required to sign an informed consent by the health care provider
- Ensuring the patient understands all information and procedures
- Validating the patient's competence to consent
- Having the patient sign the consent documents in front of you
- If the client does not understand the procedure or treatment, notify the healthcare professional
- Documentation of consent form

ALLOCATION OF SCARCE HEALTH RESOURCES

As medical costs rise and stricter cost-containment measures are put in place, the need to allocate limited amounts of health care goods or services has become an important area of concern. It is impossible to give every client what they want; the moral principle of autonomy cannot be applied in all the situations.

Ethical Dilemmas in Allocation of Scarce Health Resources

Nursing care, according to the American Nurses Association, can be considered as a "resource" or "service". To address the needs of all the patients, it must be distributed properly and equally. Nurses can use the principle of justice to try to find what is fair for the patients and family members. To reduce costs, planning the workplace design is an effort to save the health care resources. Some nurses worry that the staffing levels in their hospitals are not sufficient to provide the care they require. The shortage of nurses creates an ethical dilemma. The allocation of health resources must be balanced between caring and the recipients of caring. In today's healthcare environment, the issue of allocating scarce resources is becoming a significant ethical problem.

The current focus on controlling health care costs means that expensive services are being closely examined. The rapid rise in health care costs and shrinking public funding for primary and second-line care are two major factors that influence health care ethics. The increasing scarcity of health care resources may lead to a reduction in resources for certain programs, and possibly rationing within those programs. Health care professionals face ethical dilemmas when allocating resources. They have to deal with the clinical realities of providing more complex care using growing technologies and treatment methods.

■ CONFLICTS CONCERNING NEW TECHNOLOGIES

In the past, a medical record was information that was written on paper to be used for research, financial, legal, and clinical purposes. However, accessibility was its biggest drawback. It was only accessible to one person at a time. Because it was manually updated, its completion took anywhere from 1 to 6 months. Even today, the purpose of electronic media documentation is still to support patient care. An electronic medical record (EMR), or electronic health record (EHR), is a digital record that contains a patient's details (including their history, investigations, and treatment). EHRs are being used by hospitals and nurses because they have many advantages over traditional paper records. Producing legible records helps to reduce the risk of incorrect prescriptions, doses, and procedures. EHRs increase access to healthcare, improve quality, and reduce costs.

Ethical Dilemmas Concerning New Technologies

Health informatics is the study and analysis of health care information and communication. This field has been greatly affected by the increased use of computers and the internet by both patients and clinicians in recent years. Many practices now use electronic medical information (EMRs) as well as computerized provider order entry (CPOE). Patients are often able to search the internet for health information. In many developing countries, electronic health records (EHRs) are being increasingly implemented. This is a vital component of modern health care because it can improve the quality and cost effectiveness of healthcare. There are many risks associated with technology, making it a serious challenge to ensure that information is safe. Despite its growing utility and enthusiasm for its adoption, little attention is being paid for ethical questions that may arise.

Autonomy is compromised when confidential patient information is made public without authorization or consent and security breaches can threaten privacy. Health care workers have a legal and moral obligation to respect patient privacy and confidentiality. To prevent privacy breaches, electronic records and associated systems must be monitored and secured. Patients may hide information if they are not confident in the security of their data. Their treatment could be compromised as a result.

The EMR, which promises to be the platform that allows patients to access new functionality and services, can be a great tool yet sensitive too. Data transfer can lead to data loss or destruction. This raises questions about the accuracy and reliability of the data base, which is used for patient care decisions. Medical identity theft is a growing problem. EHRs can be used to increase patient safety, decrease healthcare errors, and improve public health. Concerns have been raised regarding the reliability and accuracy of the electronic health records. Improper use of options like "cut and paste" can lead to inaccurate representations of patient's current condition. This is unacceptable as it increases risk for patients, and also increases liability for clinicians. EMRs have many benefits but the future of healthcare requires that they are properly managed to overcome the risks.

WHISTLEBLOWING

Whistleblowing is primarily concerned with drawing attention to and exposing unlawful or immoral behavior by others. This is a form of ethical behavior that adheres to the principles of nonmaleficence and honesty. Although nurses are required to "blow the whistle" on inept health care professionals, many are hesitant as there are risks associated with whistle blowing. Unfortunately, the nurse may not be able to fulfill their ethical obligation to disclose unethical behavior because they fear reprisal and want to safeguard their colleagues at the same time.

Huston (2010), states that whistle blowing can be divided into two categories.
1. Internal whistleblowing which is occurring in an organization.
2. External whistleblowing refers to reporting outside of the organization such as to the media or elected officials.

Haddad (1999), identified some of the questions one should ask when reporting incompetent or unethical behavior.
- Has wrongdoing caused (or is it likely that it will cause) serious damage?
- Does the nurse have the competence to judge the wrongdoing?
- Is all necessary information available before you draw judgment.
- Has the nurse confirmed the information with other people?
- Has every available resource inside the organization been put toward finding a solution to the problem?
- Will reporting the issue likely rectify the wrongdoing or avoid future harm?
- Is the potential harm caused by whistleblowing less severe than that caused by wrongdoing?

Ethical Dilemmas in Whistleblowing

One example of whistleblowing by nurses is to report about the abuse faced by the patients during the course of treatment. It is interesting that even though most people want wrongdoing and corruption to be reported it is often seen with suspicion. Whistle-blowers can be considered disloyal, or face repercussions, even if their whistle blowing was done with the best intentions. Huston (2010), suggests that "nurses, as healthcare professionals, have a responsibility for uncovering, openly discussing, and condemning shortcuts which may threaten the clients they care for." Yet, many cases have been closed. It is not possible to change the situation or solve the problem by whistle-blowing. It requires a great sense of right and wrong, as well as the commitment to follow a problem until it is resolved. Nurses should consult their professional mentors or professional association before proceeding for whistle-blowing.

ISSUES RELATED TO BEGINNING OF LIFE

Because ethical issues related to life and births are often complicated, they also carry the additional burden of our personal values. Nurses must try to follow the code of ethics while dealing with such issues. Stages of beginning of life have been depicted in **Figure 6.1**. Some important issues which have been discussed in this chapter are as mentioned underneath.

Abortion

Abortion (the termination of a pregnancy before the fetus is viable) is a controversial topic that generates controversy in all settings. Medically, miscarriage and abortion refer to the termination a pregnancy before the fetus can survive outside the uterus. Many babies born as young as 24 weeks old can survive and go home with the help of technology and neonatal care. Abortion is a topic that evokes strong emotions. Because of its ethical, legal, and social implications, abortion affects everyone in some way. The issue of abortion is strongly supported or opposed by many people. Abortions could be spontaneous, which happens intentionally and it could be elective induced abortion following Medical Termination of Pregnancy (MTP Act-2021 (amended) of the country.

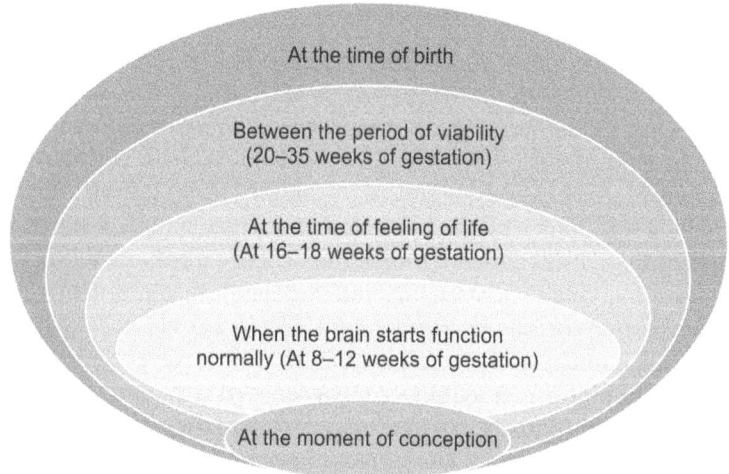

Fig. 6.1: The stages of the beginning of life.

Abortion Debate

The abortion debate is centered on two fundamental issues:

- ❖ When life begins and who has the right to choose? The opponents of abortion believe that life begins at conception and therefore abortion is an act of killing.
- ❖ Those who support abortion argue that the fetus is not human until it is able to live independently of the mother (i.e., the age of viability which is approximately 20 weeks).

Supreme Court's recent ruling issued on September, 28, 2022 stated that the distinction between married and unmarried women under MTP Act is arbitrary and all women have autonomy to exercise their rights regarding safe and legal abortion up to 24 weeks of gestation.

Deontologically, abortion is a fundamental conflict between rights. A woman's rights of privacy, self-determination, freedom of choice, and autonomy are all at stake. The other side to the abortion dilemma is that of the fetus's rights to life. Some people believe that it is against the law to take a human life casually or intentionally. The most fundamental right is life. Without it, there are no rights. In most cases, the right of life is the most important and absolute of the rights. Laws regarding abortion are constantly changing and being challenged. Ethical opinions are constantly changing and the debate continues. It includes rights of women as well as rights of the unborn. This adds to its complexity.

Ethical Dilemmas in Abortion

These conflicting rights should be weighed against one another when trying to solve the morality and ethics of abortion. Nurses are often asked to assist clients in making decisions about abortion. As often as possible, they may be asked to assist with the actual procedure. Before they assist with these procedures, and to make the best decision in the abortion dilemma, nurses need to examine their values and their perceptions of their roles. Should a nurse advocate for a client? How can a nurse not influence a woman's decision to have an abortion? A nurse can legally and ethically refuse to help with abortions. The nurse must remember, as in any ethical dilemma, that the client needs competent and high-quality care, regardless of her personal moral convictions.

The following ethical points should be kept in mind while involved in abortion:
- There is a clear and justified indication
- Provide information to clients about the stages and viability of the fetus as well as methods of abortion.
- Get informed and written consent.
- Maintain confidentiality
- Be kind and compassionate

Substance Abuse During Pregnancy

Substance abuse disorders in pregnant women continue to be a major public concern. They pose a risk to their child's development and place socioeconomic burdens on society through increasing demand for social and medical services. It is not surprising that drug addiction during pregnancy has been linked to many brain disorders. Untreated drug abuse/addiction during pregnancy often occurs in conjunction with poor nutrition and prenatal care. This increases the likelihood of obstetric complications as well as disrupting the developmental processes of the fetus. The mother as well as the developing baby can suffer from the negative health effects of substance abuse. There are ongoing efforts to criminalize pregnancy substance use.

Commonly Misused Drugs During Pregnancy and their Side Effects

Methamphetamine, cocaine, and marijuana are all illegal drugs that can harm the development of a fetus. However, common over-the-counter medications, caffeine, and alcohol can also have long-term effects on an unborn child. Pregnancy drug use can also increase the risk of stillbirths, birth defects, underweight babies, and premature babies. Severe side effects in pregnant women due to use of drugs are as follows:
- Early childhood behavior problems have been shown to be caused by an early exposure to marijuana and *ganja*. Children's attention and memory can also be negatively affected by these drugs.
- Smoking marijuana can increase the risk of having a premature baby and a low birth weight in pregnant women. The child may experience developmental delays. Smoking marijuana while pregnant appears to cause withdrawal symptoms in newborns, such as crying and trembling uncontrollably.

- Early in pregnancy, the chances of miscarriage are increased by using methamphetamine or cocaine.
- Fetal alcohol syndrome (FAS) and fetal alcohol spectrum disorders (FASD) are both names for a group of problems that can be caused by drinking alcohol while pregnant. The fetal alcohol syndrome may result in facial deformities, growth limitations, and central nervous system abnormalities. Additionally, fetal alcohol syndrome can result in learning problems, attention span problems, and additional physical deficits.
- Preterm labor, low birth weight, and fussy newborns are all possible side effects of the illicit substances.
- Drug-exposed (cocaine) infants are more likely to have smaller heads, which may imply a reduced level of cognitive ability. They are also more likely to be born with cardiac or urinary system abnormalities. Unborn babies may experience strokes due to cocaine exposure. This can lead to brain damage, or even death.

Furthermore, major complications of substance abuse in pregnancy have been illustrated in **Table 6.1**.

Table 6.1: Major complications of substance abuse.

Obstetric and fetal complications associated with maternal substance abuse	❖ Placenta previa ❖ Abruptio placentae ❖ Premature rupture of membranes ❖ Spontaneous abortion ❖ Intrauterine growth retardation ❖ Premature delivery ❖ Birth defects ❖ Neonatal long-term developmental effects
Neonatal complications	❖ Congenital anomalies ❖ Neonatal medical complications ❖ Neurobehavioral changes ❖ Sudden infant death syndrome (SIDS) ❖ Neonatal abstinence syndrome (NAS) ❖ Respiratory distress syndrome

Ethical Principles Involved In Substance Abuse During Pregnancy

These ethical issues are most important in discussing how these substances affect pregnant women and their infants. Truth (honesty in disclosing plan and consequences), autonomy (the right of a person to choose whether they wish to undergo any procedure or test), justice (equal treatment of all people, regardless of race or gender), nonmaleficence (ensuring no harm from medical actions), and beneficence (pursuing best interest). These four principles are primarily focused on the woman. The last one includes the needs of both the neonate and the mother.

A core belief is that substance abuse disorder is a medical problem rather than a moral failing. Women with substance use disorders, unlike other medical issues, labelled as child abusers. This could result in their parental rights being contested. By screening and detecting patients with substance use disorders, physicians may fear they are inviting damage or family disruption. This attitude may imply that physicians should tackle this issue in the same manner as they do similar, but less serious, medical problems.

Fetal Therapy and Intrauterine Treatment of Fetal Conditions

These terms cover a wide range of medical procedures, including open surgery and pharmacotherapy. It also includes experimental procedures that are accepted treatments, as well as treatment options that aim to save fetuses from *utero* death or perinatal death. Fetal therapy cannot be performed without the informed consent of the mother or her representative. Contrary to other medical settings, informed consent for fetal treatment is unique in that the consenting person (or nonconsenting person) not only makes decisions for herself but for the fetus, which may or not survive, and/or the future child, who may or not benefit. Consent for fetal treatment is therefore always asked and given within the context of ideas about the expectant mother's responsibility.

Maternal and Fetal Conflict

The unique situation of medical ethics in pregnancy is that the fetus cannot be accessed without the intervention on the pregnant woman. While maternal and fetal interests are usually aligned in most cases, the care of the fetus depends on the care of the woman who is pregnant. Sometimes conflict can occur between maternal and fetal interest. This is called "obstetric" and "maternal/fetal conflict. These emotionally charged issues involve the protection of the rights of women as well as the best interests for the fetus, i.e., when conflict occurs between maternal and fetal interest for example, refusing to have a cesarean delivery considering fetal distress.

Ethical Dilemma in Fetal Therapy

Fetal therapy involves a complex evaluation of both the best interests for the fetus as well as the pregnant woman's health. Physicians should consider the maternal choice and assess the risk when recommending fetal treatment that has been proven effective. In limited cases where fetal therapy is effective in preventing irrevocable, substantial fetal harm while posing no risk to the woman's health or well-being, doctors should respect the decision of the mother. Without the consent of the woman, a physician should not intervene. They should also engage in communication and conflict resolution.

Ethically, the fetus can be viewed as a patient in many different ways. The lack of clarity in legal terms further confuses decision-making. According to ethics, beneficence-based obligations to the fetus should be examined in the context of the mother's autonomy and beneficence. The following questions are much relevant to this context:

- Is a fetus considered "viable" when it is not yet born?
- What is considered "serious illness or handicap?"
- Which type of "benefit" would be sufficient to justify this decision?
- What is "unlikely" in terms of morbidity and mortality of the mother or the fetus?
- Does the biological father's role in these decisions change if the spouses are unmarried?
- What happens when a mother takes decisions that are not in her unborn child's best interest?

Selective Reduction

A medical procedure called "selective pregnancy reduction" that is used to reduce multiple pregnancies, most often those that are induced through in vitro fertilization (IVF) or drug therapy. Healthy embryos may be sacrificed to increase the chance of survival or allow the mother to select the number of children she wants to have. The likelihood of multiple pregnancies increases with assisted reproductive technology. Many fetal reductions can be done after embryo transfer and in vitro fertilization, whether for social or health reasons.

Ethical Issues In Selective Reduction

- ❖ Difficult to decide on how many fetuses should be reduced and which one to select.
- ❖ Despite the fact that decisions must be founded on technical and empirical grounds, the issue of gender selection cannot be overlooked. The screening for genetic abnormalities are determining factors for deciding the number of fetuses. The problem is that such tests include information about the gender of each fetus.
- ❖ Gender selection is a complex issue. As seen in societies with a preference for males than females, widespread sex selection can have many social implications. This includes a change in the sex ratio of the population.

Responsibilities During Selective Reduction

Deontologically, physicians and nurses have a duty to care for both mother and fetus. Multiple issues must be addressed and the health care provider should provide information about the potential outcomes of various actions (e.g., fetal reduction vs. expectant management). The following factors may be considered in the case of selective fetal reduction:

- ❖ The nature and process
- ❖ Expectant management as an option
- ❖ Potential complications, e.g., complete pregnancy loss and the risks of expectant management
- ❖ The benefits of fetal reduction (i.e., reduced maternal and fetal mortality and morbidity
- ❖ Limitations of treatment
- ❖ Success and failure rates
- ❖ Post reduction management.

The decision to reduce the number or continue multifetal pregnancies and the consequences of that decision are not simple. The emotional and psychological toll that comes with making a decision based on economic, medical, or social issues adds to the complexity. It is critical not to overlook psychological consequences such as guilt or the stress of multifetal pregnancies, as well as the option of foetal reduction. These issues should be addressed with patients who are in volatile psychological states. It is not easy to manage multifetal pregnancies.

Fetal reduction is an option but should not be used to reduce fertility. The primary goal must be to prevent higher-order multifetal pregnancy.

Mandated Contraception

Commonly, protocols that require women with childbearing potential to use one or more methods of birth control during clinical drug trial enrollment are approved by the research ethics review committees. Sometimes, the method of birth control is specified (e.g., intrauterine devices or oral contraceptives). A contraceptive requirement is designed to protect the developing fetus against exposure to drugs that could harm it. It also prevents pregnancy during the trial.

Ethical Issues In Mandated Contraception

- ❖ Some argue that it is unethical to make contraceptive use mandatory for women with childbearing potential as a condition of trial participation.
- ❖ Contraception can pose health risks to women and violates women's autonomy. These risks are magnified when contraceptive use does not exist, or when there is no chance of pregnancy.
- ❖ Others believe that mandated contraception is ethically justified for women with childbearing potential. They argue that the woman should not expose potential fetuses to potentially harmful drugs.

Many research ethics review committees have policies on contraception for women participating in clinical trials. This is to balance the obligation to respect women's autonomy, well-being, and protect potential fetuses against possible research harms. All these can create another ethical issue of participation of pregnant women in clinical drug trials. On the contrary excluding pregnant women from research, results in a dangerous lack of knowledge about the safety and efficacy of drugs used during pregnancy as well as the potential harm to the developing fetus. Lyerly, Little, and Faden claim that research without pregnant women is harmful in at least four dimensions.

- ❖ There will be no evidence to support the effectiveness of medical treatment for pregnant women.
- ❖ Information about the safety and effectiveness drugs used on the fetus will not be available.

- Pregnant women will be treated poorly if they do not take the necessary drugs for their own health. They are concerned about how their unborn child will be affected by these drugs.
- Pregnant women will not be allowed to receive the occasional benefits of trial participation.

Contraceptive policies are often focused on women and not enough attention is paid to male potential harms to the fetus. For example, there is the possibility of chemicals binding to sperm causing harm to the developing fetus. It should be recommended that women who participate in research on sexual activity and are susceptible to getting pregnant be asked to stop having sex or to use a reliable method of contraception. It would be better to have access to information about family planning at a low cost or free of charge.

Fetal Injury

Unique legal and ethical issues can arise from pregnancy. Pregnant women are autonomous and have the right to make their own decisions. The fetus is not protected in most countries. Although it is possible for future children to be hurt by the actions of mothers who are pregnant, the law generally will not apply even if there is a high likelihood of harm. Yet health practitioners have a legal obligation to report potential injury, and authorities have a legal commitment to protect the child's well-being.

In Utero Harm

There are two categories of in utero injury.
1. It can be caused by the actions of third parties. Third party harm can include physical assault on a pregnant woman or the teratogenic effect of a drug that was not properly evaluated or negligently prescribed to them.
2. In utero harm may also be caused by the actions of the pregnant woman (called "gestational harm").

Ethical Dilemmas in Fetal Injury

Maternal-fetal conflict is most commonly caused by choices made by mother that pose a risk to the fetus. This includes those based on ethical or religious motivations, ignorance, self-destructive habits, or economic imperatives. Certain situations such as not getting tested for human immunodeficiency virus (HIV), going through vigorous exercise program during pregnancy, and refuse to take tetanus vaccinations can create ethical dilemmas in front of health professionals. These situations were common in the past and involved refusal to have certain invasive medical procedures such as blood transfusions or cesarean section. These cases highlight the mother's fundamental right to religious freedom and her liberty interest by refusing unwelcome treatment, as opposed to the law's interest protecting the unborn. It is important to distinguish between harmful behaviors for the fetus that are independently illegal (e.g., abuse of controlled substances) from those that are harmful and legal (e.g., drinking alcohol). Substance abuse is a problem for anyone, but it can be a problem for pregnant women too and considered as a mean of deliberate fetal injury. This act can result in fetal harm and has legal and ethical ramifications. In some situations, pregnant mothers have been sentenced to prison for endangering their fetuses through drug addiction. Prenatal drug exposure is required to be reported under many state laws. This might result in child endangerment and carelessness charges being filed against the woman. This punitive approach to prenatal injury raises ethical and legal concerns regarding how much government oversight is required to protect infant safety.

Infertility Treatment

Infertility is "a disease of the reproductive system defined by the failure to achieve a clinical pregnancy after 12 months or more of regular unprotected sexual intercourse (according to WHO). There are two kinds of infertility:
1. Primary infertility is when a couple has not had a baby.
2. Secondary infertility is when the couple has had a previous pregnancy but failed to conceive.

Primary infertility is the most common type of infertility worldwide. Up to 15% of all couples between the ages of 15 and 45 worldwide are affected by infertility. All assisted reproductive technologies (ART) include infertility treatments that involve the handling of eggs or embryos. Some of the techniques of ART are illustrated in **Figure 6.2**.

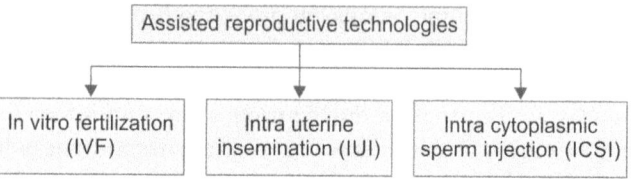

Fig. 6.2: Techniques of assisted reproductive technologies (ART).

Types of Assisted Reproductive Technologies

The three main types of assisted reproductive technologies (ART) are in-vitro fertilization, intracytoplasmic sperm injection and intrauterine insemination **(Fig. 6.2)** as detailed below:

❖ **In vitro fertilization (IVF)** is a treatment in which a female is administered with hormones to stimulate the production of eggs. In an incubator dish, the eggs are combined with sperm. The fertilized embryo is then placed back into the womb.

❖ **Intracytoplasmic sperm injection (ICSI)** involves injecting a single sperm directly into the cytoplasm of an egg. This allows to have more control over which sperm fertilizes which eggs. This method can also be performed in a laboratory, after which the fertilized egg is implanted into the womb using typical IVF techniques.

❖ **Intrauterine insemination (IUI)** is used when there is a low quality or quantity of sperms. IUI which involves the collection and insertion of healthy sperms directly into the uterus is performed when a woman is having an ovulatory period.

All of the treatments outlined above can be employed in egg donation and surrogacy. To test for genetic abnormalities, all processes can be used to do preimplantation genetic analyses. There are numerous ethical concerns surrounding infertility therapy. The American Society for Reproductive Medicine (ASRM) has issued a number of statements on the subject. Some of the concerns are as follows:

❖ **Multiple gestations:** Multiple fertilized eggs are introduced to the womb in some IVF situations to boost the odds of pregnancy. This raises the chances of several fetuses being born, which increases the risk of early births, baby health issues, and low birth weights.

❖ **Embryos:** A clinic may offer to store any fertilized eggs left over from assisted conception for future attempts. People should

think about what they want to happen to the eggs in case of death or divorce. They should also make sure to provide written instructions. Also, people should consider what they want to happen to their eggs if the clinic is unable to reach them.
- **Donor eggs/sperm or surrogacy:** One option for a couple is to have their child carried by a surrogate or donor egg or sperm. These cases require that couples talk to a lawyer or clinic about the possibility of a contract being created which outlines the rights and responsibilities of each parent and their future children.

■ **Critical Thinking**
List out the situations in which surrogacy is considered to be justifiable.

Different countries have different regulations regarding fertility treatment. Some of the examples are:
- Turkey, China, and other countries allow only married couples to undergo IVF.
- New Zealand requires a stable and nuclear family.
- The USA, Sweden, and Spain allow IVF for singles and homosexuals. If a woman is over 18 years old, she can become pregnant by IVF. Sperm from an anonymous donor will be accepted.
- The surrogacy bill 2021, Government of India banned commercial surrogacy in India.

Ethical Dilemmas in Infertility Treatment

It is a fact that ARTs, regardless how beneficial they are for medical and social purposes, can pose bioethical problems that merit consideration. These could be moral or ethical. Moral implications relate to the fact that these techniques involve the instrumental manipulation and fertilization without regard for its natural environment or the consequences that could arise. Ethical implications refer to bioethical concerns related to medical aspects of these methods. These are the concerns:
- Donor sperm and eggs can be used but the law protects anonymity
- *Embryo development time*: Many countries allow embryos to develop for several days in order to select the best embryo for implantation. However, some countries only allow embryos to be implanted early.

- *Time limit for embryo storage*: Embryos can be kept for up to 3 years in Brazil but in Spain and Canada they can be stored for an unlimited time.
- *Genetic screening and embryo selection*: In some countries, genetic screening before implantation is strictly regulated.
- *Maximum numbers of embryos per country*: Certain countries have stringent policies regarding single embryo transfer yet in some countries; the doctor's discretion is what determines the number of embryos that can be implanted.
- *Use of frozen sperm and embryos following the death of a partner*: When a male partner dies in iceland, frozen sperm is destroyed. In Belgium, however, sperm can be taken with written consent for future treatment.
- These techniques could be used for social purposes that are not related to the woman's fertility such as surrogacy and social freezing.
- Advertisements for assisted reproduction clinics might advertise success rates that are too high to attract customers.

ISSUES RELATED TO END OF LIFE

End-of-life questions can often be complex moral, legal, or ethical dilemmas. They concern the patient's vital physiological functions, medical and surgical prognosis, quality-of-life, personal values, and beliefs. Nursing can often be a witness to difficult decisions and complex situations that patients and their families face when caring for them. Although nurses are able to have their own morals, values and beliefs, sometimes they do not match the patient's wishes or values. The nurse may have internal conflict as a result of this. Some of the medical treatments and options discussed may be simple, while others will be more challenging. Nurses, regardless of the type of intervention utilized, should be able to assist patients in weighing the benefits and costs of therapy rather than focusing on the intervention itself. (Kennedy Swartz 2001). Issues related to end of life are discussed in this chapter are mentioned here:

Withholding/ Withdrawing Medical Intervention

End-of-life issues are one of the most divisive issues in contemporary bioethics. In actuality, withholding or withdrawing some forms of treatment is the simplest way to safeguard patients from the potentially detrimental effects of life-prolonging medical technology, especially when the patient's quality of life deteriorates significantly.

Withholding or removing life-sustaining interventions can be a difficult ethical and emotional minefield for everyone involved. A patient with decision-making capacity has the right to refuse or request that a medical intervention be halted, even if the decision is likely to result in death and regardless of whether the patient is terminally ill. In accordance with ethics guidelines for surrogate decision-making, where a patient lacks appropriate capacity, the patient's surrogate may deny or request that an intervention be terminated.

The cessation or reduction of medical intervention in patients is one of the problems that could arise in practice. These interventions can be minor (such as nonlife-sustaining medication) or more complicated (such as mechanical ventilation). These interventions are often stopped because the burdens outweigh the benefits for the patient. Sometimes life-sustaining therapies can prolong suffering while decreasing the patient's quality of life. These factors are often the reason patients and their families decide to discontinue medical intervention. Family members are often faced with the difficult decision of withdrawing life-sustaining treatment (or life support) from their loved ones. Advance directives are thus critical because they allow patients to make decisions about their treatment. A family member who is certain that a loved one would not want a certain medical intervention may be able to alleviate some of the stress associated with making this choice. It also helps to prevent the initiation of some life-sustaining treatments in advance, eliminating the need for a decision to withdraw such intervention, which helps to decrease the overall expenditures of unneeded medical care.

While there is an emotional difference between not beginning a treatment at all and abandoning it later in the treatment regimen, there is no ethical difference between withholding and discontinuing treatment. When an intervention no longer contributes to accomplishing a patient's care goals or desired quality of life, it is morally permissible for physicians to withdraw it.

Allow Natural Death

A newer terminology that some health care institutions are using instead of traditional DNR orders is "allow natural death". While a

DNR order prohibits the patient from initiating cardiopulmonary resuscitation, an AND order allows only comfort measures to be taken in order to manage comfort symptoms. An AND order allows the patient comfort while still allowing for natural death. Meyer (2002) proposed replacing DNR with the phrase "allow natural death" (AND), which acknowledges that death is inevitable and that the purpose of treatment in the dying phase is for the patient to be comfortable rather than to suffer unnecessarily.

Many individuals are confused by the belief that approving a DNR order grants them permission to end their loved one's life. Or they may be hesitant to comply with the instruction because they feel terrible for not assisting their loved one as much as they believe they should. Perhaps it is time to switch from do not resuscitate (DNR) to "allow natural death," a kinder, more decisive term (AND). The purpose of an order to AND is to guarantee that only comfort measures are implemented. By using AND, doctors and other medical workers are acknowledging that the patient is dying and that everything they are doing for them—including withholding nutrition and fluids — is aimed to making the dying process as painless as possible.

Allow natural death choice is a proactive, affirmative attitude that expresses the wish for people to die as calmly and naturally as possible, accompanied by their loved ones. Allowing natural death does not mean withholding or abandoning resuscitation, artificial feedings, fluids, or other procedures that would prolong a natural death. The person will continue to receive the following services in addition to the agreed-upon interventions:

- Rapid assessment and management of pain and other disturbing symptoms
- Various measures of comfort such as emotional, cultural, and spiritual assistance
- Privacy and respect for the person's dignity and humanity, as well as their family's
- If needed, monitoring of water and nutrition needs
- Oral and body hygiene.

Medical Order for Life Sustaining Treatment

These newest kinds of advance directives, also known as physician orders to life-sustaining treatment (POLST), were created to facilitate the communication of a patient's desires concerning life-sustaining therapies among healthcare practitioners and settings. Medical Orders for Life-Sustaining Treatment (MOLST) is a program that translates patient goals and preferences into medical orders in order to improve the quality-of-care patients receive at the end of life.

Medical orders for life-sustaining treatment is based on the patient, his or her health care agent or other designated surrogate decision-maker, and healthcare workers making shared, informed medical decisions. The MOLST program was developed to supplement standard advance directives and to make medical orders affecting end-of-life care more accessible to individuals with advanced chronic or catastrophic illnesses. Patients have the right to make their own healthcare decisions, including decisions about life-sustaining treatment, to convey their desires to healthcare providers, and to receive comfort care while their wishes are carried out, according to the MOLST program. The MOLST is a single document that contains a patient's goals and preferences in the areas listed here:

- Resuscitation instructions are given when a patient has no pulse and/or is not breathing.
- Follow the intubation and mechanical ventilation guidelines if the patient has a pulse and is breathing.
- Treatment recommendations
- Hospitalization and transfer in the future
- Fluids and nourishment can be artificially provided
- Antibiotics

Medical orders for life-sustaining treatment is typically used with patients who have major health problems, although it may also be appropriate for those who are older. Patients with major health problems include those with advanced, chronic, progressive illness and/or frailty (significant weakness and severe problems with personal care activities), as well as those who are likely to die or lose the abilities to create treatment decisions within a year.

Hastening Death (Principle of Double Effect)

The desire to expedite death among people who are dying is complicated, and it is a cause of debate among patients, health care providers, legal experts, and ethicists. All medical therapies include intended effects as well as the danger of unanticipated, possibly harmful side effects such as death. Total parenteral feeding, chemotherapy, surgery, and amiodarone are some examples. Individuals who voluntarily hasten death have been described as people "who have been involved in decisions about their care" who want to have control over the circumstances of their death and who may act on their desire to die with or without the support of another individual.

Many health care professionals refer to this possibility of an adverse event as a "double effect," when it is actually a secondary, unintentional consequence. The principle of "double effect" refers to some clinical decisions that have both good and unfavorable outcomes (ELNEC, 2010). A "double impact" occurs when a nurse delivers a pain medicine to relieve a patient's pain and suffering, yet the same intervention may also contribute to the hastened end. The drug will relieve the pain, but it will also lower the patient's respiration rate to levels that are unfit for life. When there is a twofold effect, the nurse or clinician should always assess the intervention's intended effect. Is the pain medicine being provided to relieve pain and suffering, or to make the patient's breathing even more difficult?

Terminal/Palliative Sedation

Terminal sedation (sometimes known as "palliative sedation") is a type of sedative used in patients nearing the end of their lives, usually as a last resort to alleviate pain (Knight and Espinosa, 2010). It sedates the patient to the point when refractory symptoms are under control. The goal is to control symptoms, and to do so, the patient is sedated to varied degrees of consciousness. The goal is not to induce or expedite death, but to alleviate pain that has not been alleviated by other means. The patient is frequently drugged to the point of unconsciousness. Palliative sedation gives patients with terminal illnesses enough medication to keep them comfortable and asleep, allowing them to be free of terrible pain and other symptoms. They lose all nourishment and hydration and usually die within a few days. Palliative sedation patients should be watched 24 hours a day to ensure proper sedation. While this type of intense monitoring can sometimes be done at home, it is primarily done at a skilled nursing facility or a hospice inpatient facility. While palliative sedation is a moral and legal choice near the end of life, it is not always a right.

Knight and Espinosa in 2010 had suggested the four criteria that a patient must meet in order to be considered for palliative sedation are mentioned here:
- ❖ The patient is suffering from a life-threatening illness.
- ❖ Severe symptoms exist that are resistant to treatment and are intolerable to the patient.
- ❖ There is a "do not resuscitate" order in place.
- ❖ The end is near (hours to days).

Although terminal sedation is often compared to assisted dying and slow euthanasia, it is not the same thing. The main difference lies in the intention or purpose of the intervention. It is not intended to cause death, but to alleviate suffering that cannot otherwise be treated. The intention of assisted dying and physician assisted euthanasia is to cause death to alleviate suffering.

Assisted Dying

Volker (2010) defines assisted dying as "an act in which an individual's suicide is deliberately hastened by the administration a drug or another lethal substance." This comprehensive term encompasses both assisted suicide and euthanasia. When a patient is given the means to commit suicide such as a deadly dose or drug, this is referred to as assisted suicide. Active euthanasia is considered when someone else does the act that ends the patient's existence. The vast majority of ethical codes issued by the major nursing organizations forbid nurses from participating in patient assisted dying.

Euthanasia and Physician Assisted Suicide

Euthanasia is a Greek term that means "good death" and is commonly known as "mercy murder."

Types of Euthanasia

The types of euthanasia are broadly classified as active euthanasia and passive euthanasia **(Fig. 6.3)** as detailed here:
- ❖ **Active euthanasia** is the act of bringing about the death of a client directly with or without consent from them. This could include administering a lethal medication to end client's suffering. No matter what the caregiver intended, active euthanasia can lead to

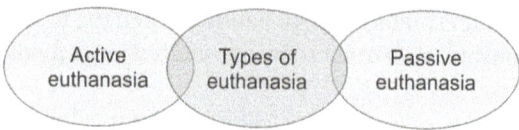

Fig. 6.3: Types of euthanasia.

criminal charges of murder. Active euthanasia can also be called *assisted suicide*, which gives clients the ability to kill themselves if requested (e.g., providing lethal doses or pills). While assisted suicide is legal in some countries, it is not permitted for clients who are terminally ill or near death. Suicide and assisted suicide remain controversial. The ANA's position on assisted suicide and active euthanasia (2013) explains that assisted suicide and active euthanasia are both in violation of the Code of Ethics for Nurses.

❖ **Passive euthanasia** [also known as withdrawing or withholding the life-sustaining therapy, and withholding or withdrawing life-sustaining treatment (WWLST)] is the removal of any extraordinary means of life support. This includes withholding attempts to revive clients (e.g., giving them "no code" status or giving them a life-support system). The client can then die due to the underlying medical condition. While assisted suicide is morally unacceptable, WWLST might be more acceptable for most people.

Nurse's Responsibility During Passive Euthanasia

Withdrawing treatment is not the same as withdrawing care. As the client's health deteriorates, nurses need to ensure that comfort and sensitive care are provided.

❖ Because it is difficult for families to stop receiving treatment, it is critical that they completely comprehend the treatment. Therefore, it is important to ensure that the antibiotics, organ transplants, and technological advancements (e.g., ventilators) can all help to extend life, but they do not always help to restore health. It is important for nurses to make family understands the treatment. They frequently have misconceptions regarding which treatments are life-saving.

❖ Clients might request that life-sustaining measures be discontinued. They may also wish to make advance directives, or designate a surrogate decision maker. Health care professionals often find it more troublesome to withdraw treatment than to start it.

Clients and their families should be kept informed. It allows them to ask questions and have a discussion about the situation. It is essential for clients to understand that they are able to change or reevaluate their decision at any time. The idea of autonomy underpins the client's freedom to refuse treatment.

> ■ **Critical Thinking**
> Euthanasia: Does any human being have the right to carry out the death of another human with or without consent from them?

Do Not Resuscitate Orders

Do not resuscitate directives specify the measures that must be withheld in the event of approaching death. Occasionally, an order to allow a natural death (AND) is issued. This indicates that only comfort measures are offered. "Nurses actively participate in assuring that appropriate and responsible interventions are used to maximize the health and wellbeing of patients under their care." This includes minimizing unneeded, unwanted or unnecessary medical treatment and patient suffering (ANA, 2015).

Cardiopulmonary resuscitation, which is required in the event of sudden death due to cardiac arrest, must be initiated by competent person. Unless the client's primary physician has issued a DNR order, agency policy permits health care staff (typically nurses) to administer CPR and other lifesaving interventions. Physician-issued DNR orders are an exception to the universal command to resuscitate. The policies that enable a DNR decision to be reached and for resolution of conflicts in decision-making are mandatory for health care agencies. A physician writing a DNR order must respect informed consent principle. The physician must have informed consent from the client and his/her guardian if the client is comatose/near death. Respecting the desires of the patient regarding resuscitation and life-support systems is an important responsibility of the nurse. It is imperative that this information is documented in the patient's records.

Patients' Right to Make Health Care Decisions

Health care facilities are required to offer clients with written information regarding their right to make care decisions. A "Do Not Resuscitate" [DNR; sometimes called "Do Not Attempt to Resuscitate" (DNAR)] order is another type of advance directive. Chest compressions, cardiac medications, and the insertion of a breathing tube are all options for CPR. A DNR is a request to not have CPR if the client ceases to breathe or is unable to sustain a heartbeat. An advance directive form can be signed at any time before or during hospitalization. In some facilities these orders are reviewed every 48-72 hours. If a terminally ill client without a DNR order tells you orally that he/she does not want to be resuscitated in a crisis, document this information and state the client's level of orientation. Notify the physician and administration, legal services, or social services of the client's wishes. Despite the fact that a DNR instruction may be contained in an advance directive, DNR orders and advance directives are legally distinct. In order for the health care practitioner to be legally protected, the client's chart should contain a documented request for a "no code" or a DNR order.

A "do not intubate" (DNI) order is frequently used in conjunction with a DNR order, which indicates that if the patient goes into cardiac arrest, they do not want to be intubated with a breathing tube. Compressions of the chest and the administration of cardiac medicines may still be used.

Protection for Nurses in Do-Not-Resuscitate

Every hospital should have a policy that describes what is expected regarding a client's medical condition in order to issue a DNR. Reordering a DNR order must be done after it has been reviewed and evaluated. Different facilities may have different review times. It is important for nurses to know if there are any laws that govern who can authorize a DNR order for incompetent clients who are no longer able. Many hospitals have policies and procedures that outline what should be done and who clients are eligible for DNR orders. American Nurses Association (ANA), published a position statement regarding nursing care and DNR orders. Position statement emphasizes the importance of nurses talking with clients and families about DNR decisions to ensure that they are fully informed before making the decision.

This includes discussing the risks and benefits of long-term treatments, comfort measures that are available, the effects and consequences of symptom palliation and understanding that aggressive technology can be withheld if it is not in the best interests of the client or his/her family. To be ethical, any decision regarding a DNR must be made based on the client's right to make their own decisions. Nursing staff face many legal challenges when dealing with conflicting or confusing DNR orders. It can be hard to interpret DNR orders that have been limited such as "do not revive except for medication and defibrillation", or "no CPR and intubation". This is especially true if there is a medical malpractice case.

ISSUES RELATED TO PSYCHIATRIC CARE

The largest group of health professionals caring for patients in the psychiatric care field is the nurses. They are able to provide quality care and manage the unique challenges associated with this patient population. This requires that nurses are educated in nursing to understand not only the many roles of psychiatric nurse but also the unique challenges and difficulties involved in caring for mentally ill patients. Some of the ethical issues encountered while caring for mentally challenged patients are discussed here.

Non-compliance to Treatment

One of the greatest problems in psychiatry is nonadherence or noncompliance to the treatment. In order to increase patient compliance and care, clinicians, and family members of patients may disguise medication in food and drink so it cannot be identified by the individual taking the drug. This practice is known as *covert/ surreptitious medication*. It is only for people who cannot consent to treatment. The use of drugs in food or drink is a widespread technique in the treatment of mentally ill individuals.

Covert medication can have major effects on the legal and ethical aspects of a patient's competence, autonomy, and understanding. The following are the ethical questions relevant to this context:
❖ Does an adult who is not able to comprehend the implications of a prescribed medication have the right to be informed?
❖ Is it the patient's right to be told about adverse effects and how they relate to the medication?

Legal Issues in Covert Administration of Medications

Covert/surreptitious administration is ethically regarded as a breach in trust by the doctor and the family members who are administering the drugs. Modern ethical practices do not permit covert medication. Treatment without consent is legal only when common law or statute allows it. It is a unique feature of psychiatry that patients are placed completely under the care and supervision of their treating doctors.

Violation of Ethical Principles in Covert Medications

The most important ethical principles regarding the use of concealment medication include autonomy, justice, and beneficence as well as respect for people. Patients who are autonomous can be considered to have the ability to make their own decisions. While autonomy is an essential principle of health care, it must also be balanced with the need to ensure public safety, ideals and duties of beneficence, and care giving.

Restraints or Seclusion

Restraints are usually used in psychiatry to refer to leather straps that are used for restraining the extremities of an individual who is out of control or poses a risk to their physical safety or psychological well-being. The Joint Commission, which accredits health care organizations, has created particular guidelines for the use of restriction and seclusion. The Joint Commission (2010) provides the following examples of existing standards:

- No matter when the order expires, seclusion or restraint will be ended as soon as possible.
- Orders for seclusion or restraint must be renewed, unless the state law is less restrictive, every 4 hours for adults over 18, every 2 hours for children age 9–17, and every hour for younger children under 9 years. These time limits allow orders to be renewed for up to 24 hours consecutively.
- Within one hour of instituting seclusion or restraint, a physician or clinical psychologist must conduct an in-person assessment. This assessment may be performed by qualified registered nurses or physician assistants, but the physician must approve.

- ❖ Staff must monitor patients who are being held and isolated simultaneously by using audio or video equipment placed near them.
- ❖ The staff who work with patients to restraining or seclude them are trained to monitor their physical and psychological wellbeing, including respiratory and circulatory health, skin integrity, and vital signs.

Seclusion or restraints are sometimes necessary for some mental disorders. This is because they can cause an individual to act out violently or become very agitated. A client is placed in a controlled environment to address a medical emergency. This can often mean that a client is placed in a room with protective surrounding.

Types of Restraints

- ❖ *Physical restrains*: The use of mechanical devices to restrict movement by the client is called *physical restraint*. These devices are used to protect the client from harm and must be monitored closely. These devices can be padded with leather or cloth that are worn around the wrist, ankles, and waist. It must be remembered that staff should not use restraints as punishment or convenience. They must try other methods to reduce agitation such as verbal intervention (talking down) and chemical restraints (tranquilizing medicine). If these measures fail to work, mechanical restraints can be used.
- ❖ Chemical restraints (mainly psychotropic drugs such as sedatives) are employed to control hyperactive behavior in disturbed clients and prevent them from needing physical restraints.

These measures are used only when verbal interventions or other less restrictive treatment options have failed or are unavailable. Nurses must attempt to calm down aggressive behavior before resorting to these methods. Sometimes the environment or other clients are the ones that have triggered the aggressive behavior. This situation may be resolved by:
- ❖ Moving the client to another part of the unit.
- ❖ Monitoring the client's behavior in seclusion or restraint is imperative. They must be stopped if they are found to be ineffective or if the client shows signs that he has regained control.

Legal Implications During Restraints and Seclusion

The legal implications for the use and abuse of restraint and seclusion are described here.

- ❖ Restraints are only legal if they are required to safeguard the client and others. The nurse may employ restraints if a client is violent or in imminent danger.
- ❖ Inappropriate use of force to restrain clients can be considered assault and battery. The nurse should always try for confining techniques before proceeding with restraints.
- ❖ The nurse must then obtain an order from the doctor. A physician must approve any restraints or seclusion. Documentation is required for clients under restraints.

> ■ **Critical Thinking**
> During emergency situations, which type of restraints are found to be ethically justifiable? Physical or chemical restraints?

Refusal to Food

Hospitalized patients suffering from mental illness are more likely to refuse food. If left untreated, it can lead to death. It can lead to an emergency situation in severe cases. It can be a long term issue that becomes ingrained and difficult to change. Paranoid delusions or persecutory beliefs about food and poisoning can lead to food refusal in schizophrenia patients. A reduced desire to restrict or stop eating and binging is associated eating disorders. Refusing to eat can lead to an electrolyte imbalance and nutritional deficiencies in clients with anorexia nervosa. Poor nutrition can lead to seizure risk for patients who refuse to eat. Food refusal is positively associated with avolition, mannerisms, and posturing (as in catatonic schizophrenia). This could lead to new psychotic symptoms in the postictal or interictal phases of the seizure.

To prevent starvation, spoon feeding, tube feeding, and intravenous nutrition may be necessary. These are temporary interventions that should be stopped when the patient resumes their oral intake. In the treatment of patients with psychiatric disorders who refuse to eat, there are also ethical, legal, and social considerations. Patients who felt they had adequate support are less likely to refuse food. It is therefore necessary to have a multifaceted approach for the treatment of mental and physical health.

■ CHAPTER HIGHLIGHTS

- ❖ When two or more of the ethical principles are at odds, there is an ethical dilemma.
- ❖ Conflict can occur between maternal and fetal interest. This is called "obstetric" and "maternal/fetal conflict".
- ❖ Do not resuscitate (DNR) orders are legally separate from advance directives.
- ❖ In India if a woman is over 18 years old, she can become pregnant by IVF.
- ❖ Substance abuse during pregnancy can increase the risk of stillbirths, birth defects, underweight babies, and premature babies.
- ❖ Covert drug delivery through food or beverages is a widespread method in the treatment of mentally ill patients, but it has ethical issues.
- ❖ Nurses who work with patients to restraining or seclude them are trained to monitor their physical and psychological wellbeing, including respiratory and circulatory health, skin integrity, and vital signs.

■ MULTIPLE CHOICE QUESTIONS

1. A disease of the reproductive system defined by the failure to achieve a clinical pregnancy after 12 months or more of regular unprotected sexual intercourse.
    a. Infertility
    b. Fertility
    c. Menopause
    d. Climacteric
2. Before treating a patient in accordance with the "code of ethics". Choose the best practice mentioned below.
    a. Tell the family members about the recommended care or treatment
    b. Obtain informed consent before treatment and record it
    c. Provide basic treatment for a patient
    d. Conscientious objections to the proposed course of treatment

3. While disclosing private information about a patient's condition or treatment, the most essential focus would be:
   a. Can convey to another healthcare practitioner who is not a part of treating team
   b. There is no obligation to convey the death-related information
   c. Convey information without taking consent from the patient
   d. Actions should not violate the fundamental rights of the patients
4. The right to decide regarding the prospective treatment plans is called as:
   a. Informed consent
   b. Nominated representative
   c. Advance directive
   d. Do not resuscitate order
5. The standard abbreviation of POLST relevant to medical orders
   a. Physician orders to life-sustaining treatment
   b. Possible omissions to life-sustaining treatment
   c. Possible orders to life-sustaining treatment
   d. Possible options to life-sustaining treatment

ANSWERS

| 1. a | 2. b | 3. d | 4. c | 5. a |

BIBLIOGRAPHY

1. Ferrell BR, Coyle N, Paice J, (Eds), Oxford textbook of palliative nursing. United Kingdom: Oxford University Press; 2014.
2. Knight P, Espinosa LA, Freeman B. 4 Sedation for refractory symptoms. Care Imminent Dye. 2015;20:61–74.
3. Lachman V. Physician-assisted suicide: compassionate liberation or murder? Medsurg Nurs. 2010;19(2):121–5.
4. Levin TT, Coyle N. A communication training perspective on AND versus DNR directives. Palliat Support Care. 2015;13(2):385-7.
5. Lyerly AD, Namey EE, Gray B, Swamy G, Faden RR. Women's views about participating in research while pregnant. IRB. 2012 ;34(4):1–8.
6. Meier PJ. Life-cycle assessment of electricity generation systems and applications for climate change policy analysis. Madison: The University of Wisconsin; 2002.
7. Rodrigues P, Crokaert J, Gastmans C. Palliative sedation for existential suffering: a systematic review of argument-based ethics literature. J Pain Symptom Manage. 2018;55(6):1577-90.
8. Scanlon C. Ethical concerns in end-of-life care. Am J Nurs. 2003;103(1):48-55.
9. Venneman SS, Narnor-Harris P, Perish M, Hamilton M. "Allow natural death" versus "do not resuscitate": three words that can change a life. J Med Ethics. 2008;34(1):2-6.
10. Volker DL. 65 Palliative Care and Requests for Assistance in Dying. Legal Eth Aspect Care. 2016. 1–8.

CHAPTER 7

Ethical Decision Making

Jaison Joseph, Rakhi Gaur

Learning Objectives

Upon completion of this chapter, the readers should be able to:
- Define the ethical decision-making process.
- Explain the significance and steps of the ethical decision-making process.
- Understand the roles and responsibilities of the ethical committee.
- Discuss ethical decision making models.
- Describe issues-related encountered in decision making process.

ETHICAL DECISION-MAKING IN NURSING

Influencing patient care outcomes is a complex process. The skills and knowledge of the nurses are essential for making an ethically sound decision. Nurses can enhance their clinical expertise through updating the current literature and sharing evidence-based research. This will improve professionalism in the nursing profession and thereby enhance patient care.

Definition

Ethical decision-making is the act of evaluating and selecting the best alternative options consistent with ethical principles.

SIGNIFICANCE OF ETHICAL DECISION-MAKING PROCESS

- ***Promotes professionalism***: To reach an ethical conclusion, it should be done with respect, openness, and honesty. This process should be based on an ethical decision-making framework

supported by the evidence. It is a great way to encourage discussion among staff nurses about health care issues and other members of the team. This provides a framework for dealing with ethical issues and promotes professional growth.
- ❖ **Resolves ethical dilemma:** The process of ethical decision-making helps to address any ethical dilemma. The foundation of ethical decision-making is ethical principles and ethical theories.
- ❖ **Promotes advocacy regarding patient's rights:** The nurse's role as the patient's advocate includes interacting with the patient and facilitating their desires and needs. However, patient advocacy is largely influenced by the power of a nurse to make ethical decisions in her care. Establishing positive and cooperative professional relationships with other healthcare team members is a significant step toward an ethical decision-making process.

■ THE PROCESS OF ETHICAL DECISION MAKING

Nursing is a problem-solving profession. Nurses are by definition problem solvers. The nursing process is one of their most important tools. The nursing process is a step-by-step method of solving problems that affect client's health and well-being. While nurses are trained to deal with client's psychological and physical needs, they often feel inept when it comes to ethical issues. If nurses are taught and practice ethical decision-making, they can develop the skills needed to make ethical decisions in any setting.

Clinical judgment is the ability to make sound decisions. After collecting data and analyzing the relationships between them, nurses form nursing judgments. Then, they take appropriate action to fix the problem. The main goal of the ethical decision-making process is to decide right and wrong for ensuring the best outcomes for the patients. Nurses need to be able to identify their values and understand the steps of ethical decision-making that could be used when making ethical decisions.

Ethical Decision-making Process: Steps

A process for ethical decision-making allows nurses to address key ethical questions and organize their thinking more sequentially and logically. The ethical decision-making process in nursing is based on the

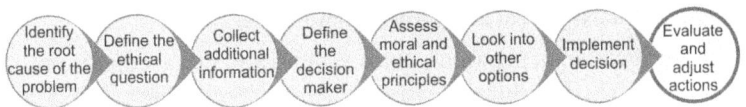

Fig. 7.1: Steps in the ethical decision-making process.

nursing process. The steps involved in the ethical decision-making process are described here **(Fig. 7.1)**:

Step 1: Define the ethical question:
It is essential to identify the key component of the ethical question relevant to the problem. It is important to distinguish the ethical problem in various aspects such as scientific basis and possible prognosis. Sometimes, social problems that arise from the conditions of a country, state, or community can also be confused with ethical questions. Therefore, these should be considered while formulating questions to address ethical issues.

Step 2: Collect additional information:
While the types of information required to solve the problem may vary, it is important to obtain all relevant information. In the decision-making process, it is possible to consider demographic data such as age, ethnicity, religious preference, education, economic status, and other information. It is important to consider the role of family members and other support networks. Further, the patient's preferences must be considered as a priority while making the decisions.

Step 3: Define the decision maker:
The patient is the primary decision-maker in determining the plans for his treatment. However, in certain circumstances, patients may not be competent to make decisions such as those who are comatose or mentally ill. In such situations, the primary caregiver or a nominated representative can be the decision maker. A nominated representative can be a family member, doctor, nurse, social worker, and other professionals who have close contact with the patient. It is important to examine the role of the nurse. The nurse may not have to make any decisions; instead, their role is to give additional information and support the decision-maker.

Steps 4: Assess moral and ethical principles:

The clarification of personal values, beliefs, and moral convictions is the key step in the ethical decision-making process. The professional code of ethics and ethical principles can act as a guide for the decision-making process. All these must be examined closely to determine if there are any ethical or moral violations for the patient or health care provider.

Step 5: Look into other options:

Once the alternatives to ethical decisions have been identified, it is necessary to predict the outcome of each option. This allows the nurse to choose the most appropriate option for her particular situation. It is important to consider the long-term and short-term consequences of each option.

Step 6: Implement the decision:

After selecting the best alternative, the next step is to implement the decision. It is important to pay close attention to the responses of the family and all members of the healthcare team. Further, it is the role of the nurse to maintain regular, accurate communication with the team and all the family members.

Step 7: Evaluate and adjust actions:

An evaluation of an ethical decision is a way to assess the decision and provide a foundation for future ethical decisions. It may be possible to change the plan or use another option if outcomes are not what were expected. The evaluation further helps to plan subsequent ethical interventions or training of the health professionals.

Ethical Decision-making Process: Models

The process of ethical decision-making can be better understood in the form of an ethical decision-making model. These models are used in making ethical decisions and are appropriate for practitioners of all levels and can be used in a variety of situations. The five steps of the model relatively resemble the steps of the nursing process. Assessment, problem identification, identification of alternative decision, implementation, and evaluation.

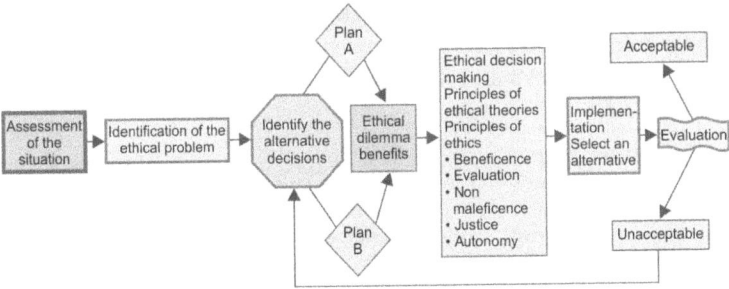

Fig. 7.2: Ethical decision-making model.

A schematic representation of this model is presented in **Fig. 7.2** and the explanation of each step is discussed here:

1. **Assessment:** *Accurate* understanding of the ethical dilemma is the initial step that provides a framework and justification for the collection of subjective and objective data.
2. **Problem identification:** The identification and evaluation of the problem causing the ethical dilemma are the most critical and the second step. This involves the evaluation of the possible course of action for the identified problems
3. **Identification of alternative decisions:** This step involves the systematic exploration of the benefits and consequences of each alternative action. The selection of the best alternative is based on the understanding of ethical principles and ethical theories. The process of evaluating the positives and negatives of an alternative action might be based on the consequences of action (utilitarianism) or based on rules and regulations (Kantianism) or avoiding actions that cause harm (non-maleficence).
4. **Implementation:** This step involves implementing the most ethical/least unethical course of action.
5. **Evaluation:** The final step involves the evaluation outcomes of the selected action. If the outcome is unacceptable, the risk and benefits of the other listed alternatives are re-examined.

Application of Ethical Decision-making Model—A Case Study

Mrs AB, a 35-year-old and the mother of three children visits a maternity clinic. She asks the nurse, to give her some information about the contraceptive measures. However, her husband is against the practice of birth control practices and prohibits distributing this type of information to her. The nurse faces an ethical dilemma while attending to Mrs AB and the process of ethical decision is depicted in **Table 7.1**.

Table 7.1: Ethical decision-making model—case study.

Assessment	Problem identification	Identification of alternative decisions	Implementation	Evaluation
A client requested information regarding contraceptive practices	A conflict exists between the client's need for knowledge, the nurse's willingness to provide it, and the husband of the client prohibiting the provision of that information	Plan A: Give the client information and risk allegations from the client's husband Plan B: Do not give the client information and compromise own moral values	Selecting the best alternative action Plan A is suggested based on ethical decision making Principles Autonomy Nonmaleficence Beneficence Justice Theories Virtue ethics Consequences Moral duty	Acceptable outcome—Maintaining the recommended contraceptive schedule. Unacceptable outcome—noncompliance with the recommended contraceptive schedule resulting in pregnancy

ISSUES IN ETHICAL DECISION MAKING

There are some situations in which the ethical decision-making process becomes troublesome for the nurses. These situations can pose legal and ethical issues if they are not properly addressed. Ethical decision-making demands special attention according to certain issues that might encounter during the decision-making process. Some of the issues in ethical decision-making are listed here:

❖ **Issues concerning consent:** Every therapeutic procedure usually involves some degree of risk, discomfort, or sacrifice from the patient's side. However, when subject's capacities to make decisions are impaired, there arises a conflict to provide informed consent. For example, clients with major mental illnesses lack adequate decision-making capacity. In such conditions, a nominated representative can provide consent on behalf of the patient.

- ❖ **Issues concerning confidentiality:** Practicing confidentiality is necessary to protect the health of patients and uphold people's faith in the healthcare delivery system. However, sometimes breaching confidentiality is unavoidable but not necessarily unethical. These include the verbalization of the commission of a violent act, human immunodeficiency virus (HIV) positive status, etc., warrants the need to disclose the matter to the concern.
- ❖ **Issues concerning rights of patients:** The client's right to refuse the medication possesses certain issues in the ethical decision-making process. This is of most importance in certain areas such as psychiatric settings, oncology settings, etc. However, if the client has a reasonable prospect of benefiting from the prescribed medication or the client it seems to be dangerous to himself or others, the physician may prescribe the medication without seeking the client's rights.

ETHICS COMMITTEE

Healthcare professionals have a responsibility to determine and resolve the complex ethical dilemmas that they face. However, they should not take such decisions on their own or without considering the viewpoints of others. Leaders, employees, and stakeholders can all benefit from a formal decision-making process when confronting ethically challenging situations. Healthcare organizations need to have resources such as ethics committees, consultation services, and written policies, procedures, and frameworks that will assist them in making ethical decisions. These guidelines and organizational resources will allow for timely and thoughtful evaluation of the best interests of patients, families, caregivers, and the community.

Research Ethics Committees

Research ethics committees are multidisciplinary, independent groups of individuals appointed to review biomedical research protocols involving human beings to help ensure in particular that the dignity, fundamental rights, safety, and well-being of research participants are duly respected and protected. The research ethics committee is usually appointed by institutions or by regional or national authorities.

Basic Responsibilities of Research Ethics Committees

- To protect the dignity, rights, and well-being of potential research participants.
- To ensure that universal ethical values and International Scientific Standards are expressed in terms of local community values and customs.
- To assist in the development and the education of a research community responsive to local health care requirements.
- To promote ethical standards in health research.
- To develop methods to promote consistency and prevent duplication of effort.

In nutshell, the primary role and responsibility of the research ethics committees is to ensure that biomedical research is conducted ethically.

Research Ethics Committee—Members

A research ethics committee is multidisciplinary and multisectoral in composition.

The number of persons in an ethics committee should be kept fairly small (8–12 members). It is generally accepted that a minimum of five persons are required to form the quorum without which a decision regarding the research should not be taken. The members should be a mix of medical/nonmedical, scientific, and nonscientific persons including lay persons to represent the different points of view.

The members may be as follows:

- Chairperson
- One-two persons from the basic medical science area
- One-two clinicians from various institutes
- One legal expert or retired judge
- One social scientist/representative of a nongovernmental voluntary agency
- One philosopher/theologian
- One lay person from the community
- Member Secretary

Roles and Responsibilities of the Ethics Committee in Clinical Decision Making

There are some roles and responsibilities for the ethics committee in the clinical decision-making process:
- Clinical studies should not include pregnant or nursing mothers unless they are intended to safeguard or improve the health of pregnant or nursing women, fetuses, or nursing infants.
- The permission of the parents or guardian must be obtained for procedures involving children. The decision of the child to decline study participation must always be respected.
- Prisoners with serious illnesses or those who are at high risk for serious illnesses should not be denied access to experimental medicines, vaccines, or other treatments that have the potential to be therapeutic or preventive.
- The doctor must not use any novel diagnostic or therapeutic procedure if it has the potential to harm lives, deteriorate health
- Every patient, including those in any control group, should be guaranteed the best available diagnostic and treatment approach in any medical study.
- The doctor-patient relationship must never be harmed by a patient's unwillingness to take part in a study.

Roles and Responsibilities of the Ethics Committee in Research

The ethics committee has a specific role in making a valid decision for conducting the biomedical research process.

Role of Research Ethics Committees: Before Conducting Research

The primary role of a research ethics committee is the accurate ethics review of research proposals. The ethics committee evaluates the research proposals in two aspects.
- Ethical implications of the research results: In this, the potential benefits and consequences of the research in local and societal contexts are evaluated.

❖ Ethical implications of the research on study participants: In this, the research participant's perspectives such as safeguarding their rights, dignity, safety, and well-being are evaluated. The ethics committee further assesses the possible ethical issues involved in the research project based on the ethical principles such as benefit-risk assessment, scientific design, and conduct of the study, payment for participation, protection of privacy and confidentiality, qualification of researchers and adequacy of study sites, selection and recruitment of participants, disclosure of conflict of interest, plans for medical management, and compensation for study related injury.

Role of Research Ethics Committees: During the Research

The research ethics committee makes necessary follow-ups and informs the researchers to maintain an appropriate record of the conduct of research projects that they have approved. This is ensured by giving the obligation of submitting the report on a regular or annual basis. The research ethics committee will advise researchers to make protocol changes, temporarily halt the study, or terminate it in the event of unacceptable results.

Role of Research Ethics Committees: After Research

This is the role that starts when the research has been completed according to the research protocol. Making the overall findings of the study accessible to research participants in a way that makes sense to them is a crucial responsibility. The second duty is to support accurate reporting of research data through fair and sufficient publication. In some cases, study findings, especially "negative" findings, are repressed; this biased under-reporting is not only unethical and unscientific, but it has potential risk for patients, for instance when side effects of therapies are covered up.

■ CHAPTER HIGHLIGHTS

❖ The act of making decisions is the process of selecting and considering options that will help to achieve the desired outcome.
❖ The decision-making process should be based on a sound ethical, decision-making model, using the best evidence-based-practice guidelines available.

Chapter 7: Ethical Decision Making

- Nurses must be able to use critical thinking to keep up with the rapidly changing health care system and new technologies.
- Clinical judgment is the ability to make sound decisions
- Healthcare organizations have ethics committees to assist in making ethical decisions. The primary role and responsibility of the research ethics committees are to ensure that biomedical research is conducted ethically.

MULTIPLE CHOICE QUESTIONS

1. The number of persons in an ethics committee should be kept as?
   a. 2–4 members
   b. 4–6 members
   c. 8–12 members
   d. 14–22 members
2. Which of the following are the issues in ethical decision-making process?
   a. Issues related to consent
   b. Issues related to confidentiality
   c. Issues related to the rights of the patients
   d. All of these
3. Which of the following is not a step in the ethical decision-making process?
   a. Define ethical question
   b. Define ethical decision maker
   c. Define the alternative decisions of choice
   d. Punishment of ethical violations
4. The following are the significance of ethical decision-making process
   a. Promotes professionalism
   b. Promotes patients advocacy
   c. Resolves issues related to the rights of the patients
   d. Resolves the financial burden
5. The following are the members of the research ethics committee except:
   a. Chairperson
   b. Member Secretary
   c. Political Secretary
   d. Legal Expert

ANSWERS

| 1. c | 2. d | 3. d | 4. d | 5. c |

BIBLIOGRAPHY

1. Amer AB. Understanding the ethical theories in medical practice. Open J Nurs. 2019;9(02):188–93.
2. Avasthi A, Ghosh A, Sarkar S, Grover S. Ethics in medical research: General principles with special reference to psychiatry research. Indian J Psychiatry. 2013;55(1):86–91.
3. Behera SK, Das S, Xavier AS, Selvarajan S, Anandabaskar N. Indian Council of Medical Research's National Ethical Guidelines for biomedical and health research involving human participants: The way forward from 2006 to 2017. Perspect Clin Res. 2019;10(3):108–14.
4. Bhutta ZA. Ethics in international health research: a perspective from the developing world. Bull World Health Organ. 2002;80:(2) 114-20.
5. Guillemin M, Gillam L, Rosenthal D, Bolitho A. Human research ethics committees: examining their roles and practices. J Empir Res Hum Res Ethics. 2012;7(3):38-49.
6. Klumagan CM. Recognizing Ethical Terms, Theories, and Principles. Ethical Competence in Nursing Practice: Competencies, Skills, Decision-Making. New York: Springer Publishing Company; 2016.
7. Ling TJ, Hauck JM (2016). The ETHICS model: comprehensive, ethical decision making. [Online] Available from https://www.counseling.org/docs/default-source/vistas/the-ethics-model.pdf [Last accessed December, 2022].
8. Martín-Arribas MC, Rodríguez-Lozano I, Arias-Díaz J. Ethical review of research protocols: experience of a research ethics committee. Rev Esp Cardiol (Engl Ed). 2012;65(6):525–9.
9. Masic I, Hodzic A, Mulic S. Ethics in medical research and publication. Int J Prev Med. 2014;5(9):1073–82.
10. Mathur R, Swaminathan S. National ethical guidelines for biomedical & health research involving human participants, 2017: A commentary. Indian J Med Res. 2018;148(3):279–83.
11. Mathur R, Thakur K, Hazam RK. Highlights of Indian Council of medical research national ethical guidelines for biomedical and health research involving human participants. Indian J Pharmacol. 2019;51(3):214–21.
12. Rich K, Butts JB. Foundations of ethical nursing practice. Role development in professional nursing practice, 3rd edition. Burlington: Jones & Bartlett Learning; 2014: pp. 105–22.
13. Rodger D, Blackshaw B. An introduction to ethical theory for healthcare assistants. Br J Healthcare Assist. 2017;11(11):556-61.
14. Sanmukhani J, Tripathi CB. Ethics in clinical research: The Indian perspective. Indian J Pharm Sci. 2011;73(2):125–30.
15. Stark L, Hedgecoe A. A practical guide to research ethics. The Sage Handbook of Qualitative Methods in Health Research. New York: Sage; 2010.

16. Thomasma DC. Theories of medical ethics: The philosophical structure. Military Medical Ethics. United States: Office of the Surgeon General, United States Army; 2003. pp;1:23–60.
17. Townsend MC, Morgan KI. Psychiatric mental health nursing: Concepts of care in evidence-based practice, 7th edition, FA Davis Company; 2017.
18. Vallotton MB. Council for international organizations of medical sciences perspectives: protecting persons through international ethics guidelines. Int J Integr Care. 2010;10 Suppl (5):e008.
19. World Health Organization. Research ethics committees: basic concepts for capacity-building. Geneva: World Health Organization; 2009.

CHAPTER 8

Code of Ethics and Patient Rights

Navjot Kaur, Shiv Kumar Mudgal

Learning Objectives

Upon completion of this chapter, the readers should be able to:
- Understand the code of ethics for nurses given by the International Council of Nurses (ICN) and Indian Nursing Council (INC)
- Describe the patient's rights given by the Ministry of Health & Family Welfare, Government of India.

CODE OF ETHICS

Since the beginnings of organized nursing in the mid-1800s, nurses have increasingly recognized four fundamental nursing responsibilities—to promote health, prevent illness, restore health, and relieve suffering and support a peaceful death. The nursing profession is deeply committed to upholding human rights, which include cultural rights, the right to life and personal independence, and the right to care with respect and dignity. Nursing care is provided without discrimination based on age, color, culture, physical or mental illness, race and sex, gender preference, national origin, politics, language, race, religion, spirituality, or legal or socioeconomic status of the people. Nurses collaborate with other healthcare workers and related organizations to provide seamless care by upholding certain values such as respect, empathy, caring, compassion, trustworthiness, etc.

Code of Ethics by International Council of Nurses

The International Council of Nurses (ICN) first approved a global code of ethics for nurses in 1953. Since then, it has undergone numerous revisions and reorganizations, most recently in 2021.

Purpose of the Code

❖ To define and direct ethical nursing practice within the context of the various nursing roles.
❖ To act as a guideline for the ethical decision-making process to achieve the standards of practice established by the regulatory bodies.
❖ To offer direction regarding nurse's roles, responsibilities, and professional judgment, to patients, their caregivers, and other healthcare professionals.

The International Council of Nurses Code

A framework for ethical behavior is provided by the ICN Code of Ethics for Nurses, which consists of four main components (**Fig. 8.1**).
❖ Nurses and patients or other people requiring care or services:
  ▪ Individuals, families, societies, and populations who require nursing care and services currently or in the long-term are the main responsibility of professional nurses.

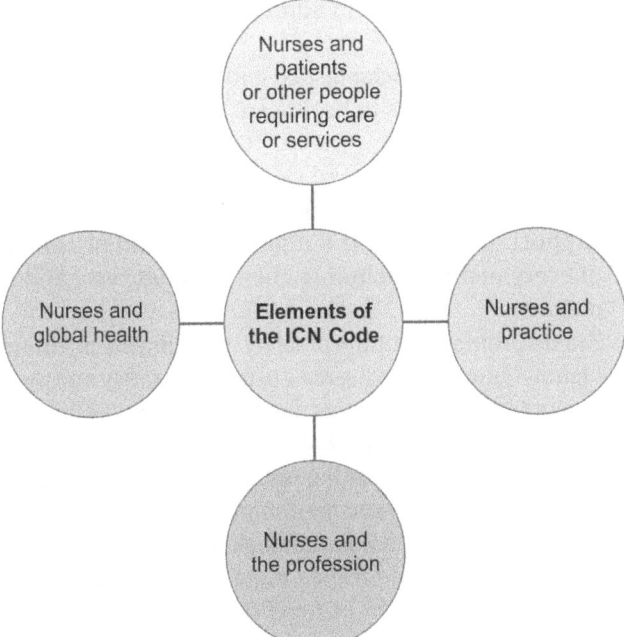

Fig. 8.1: Elements of International Council of Nurses (ICN) code of ethics for nurses.

- Nurses work to foster a culture where everyone acknowledges and respects the individual's human rights, beliefs, traditions, religious, and spiritual beliefs. Human rights encompass the rights of nurses, which must be protected and upheld.
- To establish consent for care and associated treatment, nurses ensure that the patient and family are informed in a way that is appropriate for their culture, language, cognitive skills, physical requirements, and mental condition.
- Nurses respect patient's rights to privacy, confidentiality, and the lawful collection, use, access, transmission, storage, and disclosure of personal information. They hold such information in strict confidence and only use it as necessary.
- Nurses are responsible for upholding the dignity of the nursing profession both in person and across all forms of media, including social media. This includes respecting the privacy and confidentiality of patients, as well as, the privacy and confidentiality of other healthcare professionals.
- Nurses are jointly responsible with society for launching and promoting initiatives to address the healthcare and social needs of everyone.
- Nurses promote social justice and equity in the distribution of resources, access to healthcare, and other socioeconomic facilities.
- Nurses demonstrate moral values such as fairness, kindness, attentiveness, empathy, trustworthiness, and integrity. They support and uphold the dignity and fundamental rights of every person, including clients, employees, and family members.
- Nurses promote a culture of safety in healthcare institutions by identifying and resolving risks to people's safety and providing safe practice in procedures, facilities, and environments.
- Nurses offer evidence-based, client-centered care while acknowledging and putting into practice the core values and tenets of healthcare and the promotion of health.
- Nurses make sure that technological and scientific advancements respect people's rights, dignity, and safety. Nurses make sure that care is person-centered and that artificial intelligence and devices like drones or care robots, support rather than a substitute for interpersonal relationships.

- ❖ Nurses and practice:
  - Nurses are personally accountable for ethically practicing nursing and for upholding their competence through lifelong learning and ongoing professional development.
  - Nurses uphold their ability to practice, to preserve their capacity, and to deliver high-quality, safe, and effective care.
  - Nurses are expected to practice within the boundaries of their competence as well as the legislated or licensed scope of their profession. Additionally, they are expected to exercise professional judgment when accepting or delegating duty.
  - Nurses prioritize their self-respect, health, and wellness. To accomplish this, positive practice environments, are characterized by professional recognition, education, reflection, support structures, adequate resourcing, sound management practices, and occupational health and safety.
  - Nurses always uphold ethical standards of behavior. They enhance the profession's image and the public's confidence in it. Nurses recognize and uphold personal relationship boundaries in their professional roles.
  - Nurses mentor and support the professional development of nursing students, coworkers, and other healthcare professionals by sharing their knowledge, providing feedback, and sharing their expertise.
  - Nurses act as patient advocates and uphold a practice culture that encourages moral conduct and open communication.
  - While nurses have the right to refuse participation in certain procedures or studies, they must facilitate a timely and respectful manner to ensure that patients receive services that are in line with their specific requirements.
  - Nurses uphold an individual's right to grant and revoke the authority to access their personal, health, and genetic details.
  - Nurses safeguard people, families, and societies when their health is compromised by a teammate, another person, a rule/regulation, a practice, or inappropriate use of technology.
  - Nurses actively contribute to the promotion of patient safety. When errors or near-misses happen, they promote ethical behavior, take a stand for patient safety, promote fairness, and work with others to minimize the likelihood of errors.
  - It is the responsibility of nurses to maintain data security, in order to facilitate and support ethical standards of ethical care.

- ❖ Nurses and the profession:
  - Nurses take the lead in developing and delivering appropriate professional standards for clinical practice, training, management, and research.
  - Nurses and nursing experts are spreading research-based, professional knowledge to support clinical practice based on evidence.
  - Nurses actively develop and uphold a set of core professional values.
  - Nurses, through their professional organizations, contribute to the creation of a positive and constructive practice environment in which clinical care, education, research, management, and leadership are incorporated into the practice of nursing. This encompasses safe working environments, as well as, socially and economically equitable for nurses, and that support a nurse's ability to practice within their ideal scope of practice and to provide timely, effective, and safe healthcare.
  - Nurses help to create a constructive and ethical environment within the organization by challenging unethical practices and environments. Nurses work with other nurses, other health disciplines, and relevant communities to create, conduct, and share peer-reviewed, ethically sound research and practice advancement as it relates to professional nursing care and health.
  - Nurses conduct, disseminate, and apply research that helps to improve the health of persons, families, and societies.
  - Nurses appropriately prepare for and respond to conflicts, crises, pandemics, epidemics, emergencies, and resource scarcity. Nurses and the executives of healthcare services and organizations are both accountable for the safety of those receiving care and services. This entails identifying risks, developing mitigation strategies, and putting them into action.
- ❖ Nurses and global health:
  - Nurses affirm that everyone should have the right to universal health care access because they believe that health care should be regarded as a fundamental human right.
  - Nurses defend the worth, dignity, and freedom of every person and oppose all forms of exploitation, including child labor and human trafficking.

- Nurses develop sound health policies or take the initiative in doing so.
- Nurses make important contributions to the health of the general public and work toward the realization of the Sustainable Development Goals (SDGs) established by the United Nations. (UN)
- Nurses know how important social factors are when it comes to health. They advocate for and contribute to policies and programs pertaining to them.
- Nurses collaborate, practice, and understand the need to conserve, protect, and nature as well as the health effects of environmental deterioration, such as climate change. To promote health and wellbeing, they support initiatives that limit environmentally destructive behaviors.
- Nurses promote respect for human rights, equality, and impartiality as well as the public welfare and a healthy environment in collaboration with other members of the health and social care sectors, as well as the general population, to affirm the principles of justice.
- Nurses work together around the globe to create and uphold policies and guidelines for global health.

Code of Ethics by Indian Nursing Council

1. The nurse respects the uniqueness of the individual in the provision of care.

   Nurse:
   - Cares for people without regard to their caste, creed, religion, culture, race, gender, socioeconomic background, political affiliation, or other characteristics.
   - Individualizes care taking into account the patient's values, beliefs, and cultural sensitivity.
   - Recognizes the individual's role in the family and society and encourages significant others to participate in the care.
   - Establishes and fosters a trustworthy relationship with the individual(s).
   - Recognizes the individuality of each person's response to interventions and make appropriate adjustments.

2. The nurse respects the rights of individuals as a partner in care and helps in making informed choices.

Nurse:
- Respects the right of individuals to decide their treatment by providing them with sufficient and accurate information to enable them to do so.
- Appreciates the care decisions made by an individual or individuals.
- Safeguards people against misinformation and misunderstandings.
- Advocates for special protections for those who are weaker than others (vulnerable).

3. The nurse respects an individual's right to privacy, maintains confidentiality, and shares information judiciously.

Nurse:
- Recognize the right of individuals to the confidentiality of their data.
- Keeps personal data private, unless it could put someone's life in danger, and shares information carefully.
- Obtains informed consent and ensures confidentiality whenever data is required for quality management, educational, or legal purposes.
- Restrict access to all written and electronic personal records to entitled personnel only.

4. The nurse maintains competence to render quality nursing care.

Nurses:
- Only registered nurses are allowed to provide nursing services.
- The nurse upholds care standards and works hard to deliver high-quality nursing care.
- The nurse is committed to lifelong learning and takes the initiative to confiscate any chance for self-improvement.
- Nurses value research as a tool for the advancement of the nursing profession and engage in it while upholding ethical standards.

5. The nurse is obliged to practice within the framework of ethical, professional, and legal boundaries.

Nurse:
- Adhering to the Indian Nursing Council's code of ethics and professional conduct for nurses.
- Comprehends pertinent state laws and practices in line with state law.

6. The nurse is obliged to work harmoniously with members of the health team.

    Nurse:
    - Recognize the teamwork involved in providing services/treatment.
    - Works in concert with teammates to achieve team goals and fulfill individual needs.
7. Nurse commits to reciprocate the trust invested in the nursing profession by the society.

    Nurse:
    - Maintains a high standard of personal etiquette in all interactions.
    - Exhibits professionalism in all interactions.

Code of Professional Conduct for Nurses in India

1. Professional responsibility and accountability:

    Nurse:
    - Appreciates and nurtures one's sense of worth.
    - Upholds moral standards that are commendable to the profession.
    - Fulfills obligations within the parameters of one's professional boundaries.
    - Is responsible for upholding the Indian Nursing Council's practice standards.
    - Is responsible for one's actions and decisions.
    - Is sympathetic.
    - Responsible for ensuring that current practices are continually improved.
    - Gives people enough information so they can make informed decisions.
    - Demonstrates healthy habits.
2. Nursing practice:

    Nurse:
    - Delivers services in line with established professional standards.
    - Provides physical, psychological, emotional, social, and spiritual care to all people with respect and dignity.

- Respects people and their families in the perspective of customs and culture, fostering healthy habits, and avoiding harmful ones.
- Helps people and families make autonomous decisions by presenting a factually accurate and complete picture in all circumstances.
- Encourages individuals and close family members to participate in the care
- And assures safe conduct
- When a patient's care needs exceed what the nurse is capable of handling, she consults, coordinates, collaborates, and follows-up as necessary.

3. Communication and interpersonal relationship.

Nurse:
- Develops and upholds successful relationships with people, families, and societies.
- Respects the worth of teammates and upholds healthy interpersonal relationships with them.
- Respects and encourages team members' contributions to the profession.
- Meets the needs of individuals, families, and communities in collaboration with other healthcare professionals.
- Valuing human beings.

Nurse:
- Takes the necessary steps to safeguard people from unethical conduct that is harmful.
- Thinks about pertinent information while making moral decisions that are in people's best interests.
- Encourages individuals to exercise their right to speak out on matters affecting their well-being.
- Respects and encourages personal decision-making.

4. Management:

Nurse:
- Making sure that resources are used and allocated properly.
- Supervises and teaches students and other formal healthcare workers while doing so.
- Makes decisions based on individual competency while having to accept and assign responsibility.

- Helps to create a conducive work environment to accomplish institutional goals.
- Utilizes suitable channels of communication to effectively communicate.
- Takes part in the appraisal system.
- Takes part in the assessment of nursing services.
- Takes part in policymaking while adhering to the principle of service equity and accessibility.
- Works with people to determine their needs and educates funding and policy-making organizations about resource allocation.

5. Professional advancement:

Nurse:
- Maintains respect for human rights while working to further addition in the improvement of knowledge.
- Supports the advancement of nursing practice.
- Participates in deciding and putting into practice quality care.
- Assumes responsibility for keeping knowledge and skills up to date.
- Conducts and participates in research to advance the fundamental knowledge of their field.

■ PATIENT'S RIGHTS

The 1948 Universal Declaration of Human Rights highlights the inherent worth and equality of equal rights for everyone. In the previous few decades, the notion of Patient Rights has evolved globally based on this principle. Globally, there is increasing agreement that all patients ought to have a specific set of basic rights. To put it another way, the patient has a right to a certain level of protection from healthcare professionals, caregivers, and the government, which has been outlined in many communities and countries as Charters of Patient's Rights.

In India, there are many laws about patients' rights that are written in different places. For example, the Constitution of India, Article 21, the Indian Medical Council (Professional Conduct, Etiquette, and Ethics) Regulations 2002, the Consumer Protection Act of 1986, the Drugs and Cosmetics Act of 1940, the Clinical Establishment Act of 2010 and its rules and standards, as well as, several decisions made

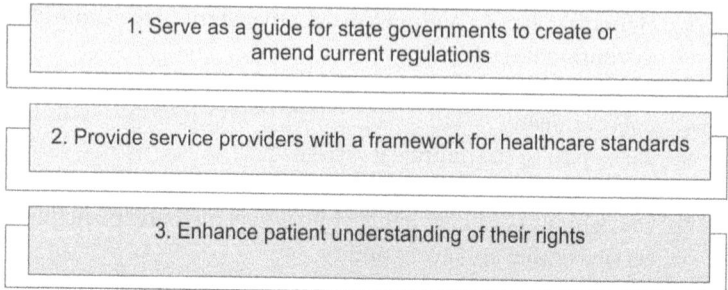

Fig. 8.2: Aims of the charter of patient rights.

by the Honorable Supreme Court of India and decisions made by the National Human Rights Commission of India, are all related to patients.

The Ministry of Health and Family Welfare published the first "Charter of Patient Rights" (the "Draft Charter") on August 30, 2018, which outlines the fundamental rights of Patients. The National Human Rights Commission (NHRC) adopted this Draft Charter, which was influenced by international charters and guided by national needs. The Charter's aims are presented in **Figure 8.2**. The Draft Charter outlines the following 17 fundamental rights for patients:

1. **Right to Information:** Each patient has the right to sufficient, pertinent information regarding the type, etiology, provisional or final diagnosis, suggested tests and treatments, and potential side effects. To be explained in a way that they can understand and in a language they already know. The concerning physician has a responsibility to make sure that the patients are provided with the information straightforwardly and understandably, either directly by the doctor or through one of his or her trained helpers. All the patients and their authorized carers have the right to receive actual, realistic information about the anticipated treatment cost. Hospital management must send this information to the patient and his/her caretaker. Any additional costs owing to a change in the patient's health state or therapy should be communicated in writing. After treatment, the patients have a right to get a detailed statement, an explanation of the bill(s), and payment receipt(s).

Every patient and caretaker for them has the right to identity disclosure and official position of all caregivers who are taking care of them, as well as the identity of the health care provider who is principally accountable for their treatment. The hospital administration must routinely deliver this information in writing with an acknowledgment to all patients and carers.

2. **Right to Records and Report:** Access to originals and photocopies of the case file, inpatient record, and investigative reports is a right granted to each patient or his carer. This may be provided after paying photocopying fees or photocopying by patients at their cost. The patient's family members or caretakers are entitled to receive the discharge summary or death summary (if the patient died) along with the original investigation reports. These records and reports must be provided by the hospital administration, and they must also give instructions to the accountable hospital employees so that they are always complied with in full.

3. **Right to Emergency Medical Care:** The Supreme Court has ruled that all institutions, both public and private, are required to offer basic emergency services to the injured people and they have a legal right to such care. This service must be given to the patient regardless of their ability to pay and must be begun without requiring payment or an advance.

4. **Right to Informed Consent:** Each patient has the right to informed consent before any diagnostic procedure or treatment that entails substantial risks. The responsibility for ensuring that all doctors understand how to obtain informed consent rests with the hospital administration, who must also ensure that a pertinent policy is in place and that patients receive consent forms that include information on how to obtain informed consent. The primary treating physician is responsible for outlining to the patient and any caregivers involved in their care the main risks associated with the procedure. Only when the patient or caregiver has given written consent, or in a manner described under the Drugs and Cosmetic Act Rules of 2016, may the physician proceed with the potentially harmful examination or treatment.

5. **Right to Confidentiality, Human Dignity, and Privacy:** Each patient has the right to privacy, and professionals are obligated to strictly enforce confidentiality regarding their health status and treatment regimen unless it is necessary to share this information to protect others or for reasons of public health. During a medical exam with a male doctor, a woman has the right to bring another woman with her. The management of the hospital is the one who is responsible for ensuring that there are female attendants available for female patients. The management of the facility is responsible for ensuring that all staff members treat patients with respect at

all times and maintain their dignity. All information related to the patient should be protected in a secure facility and protected from data leakage and theft.

6. **Right to Second Opinion:** All patients have a right to consult with an appropriate clinician of their choice for a second opinion. The hospital administration must uphold the patient's right to get another opinion and give all needed information to the patient's attendants without further charge or inconvenience. The hospital administration is responsible for ensuring that a patient/caregiver's seeking a second opinion does not compromise the quality of services delivered by the same facility while the patient is under its treatment. Any form of discriminatory action taken by the hospital or healthcare professionals will be considered a violation of human rights.

7. **Right to Transparency in Rates and Care According to Prescribed Rates wherever Relevant:** Both patients and family members have a right to knowledge about the prices the hospital will charge for each type of treatment given and the amenities available, which should be displayed prominently and described in a brochure. At the time of payment, they are entitled to receive a detailed bill that lists each item. The Hospital/Clinical Establishment would be responsible for prominently displaying key rates in both the local and English languages, as well as making the entire schedule of rates available to all the patients and family members. Each patient has the right to purchase necessary medications under the Indian Pharmacopoeia, as well as implants, at prices set by the National Pharmaceutical Pricing Authority (NPPA) as well as other pertinent governing bodies. Each patient has a legal right to get medical treatment within the price range set by the Central and State Governments from time to time, when applicable, for procedures and services. The affordability of the patient's right to choose cannot, however, be used to deny any patient their option in terms of medications, devices, or standard treatment recommendations. Every clinical facility and hospital has a responsibility to make sure that patients receive the essential medicines, implantable devices, and facilities/care at rates that do not exceed the decided price/the maximum retail price printed on the packaging, according to the Government of India and the World Health Organization.

8. **Right to Nondiscrimination:** Every individual who seeks medical care is entitled to get medical care regardless of their conditions

and diseases, including their human immunodeficiency virus (HIV) status or any other medical problem, religion, class, race, gender, age, sexual identity, language background, or geographically or socioeconomic origins. It is the responsibility of the hospital administration to ensure that no patient is subjected to discriminatory behavior or treatment. The hospital administration must periodically orient and train all its physicians and personnel on the subject.

9. **Right to Safety and Quality Care According to Standard:** In the hospital setting, each patient has a right to feel safe and secure while they are there. They have a right to get treatment in a setting that is clean enough, has infection control measures in place, has access to safe drinking water that complies with the Bureau of Indian Standards (**BIS**)/Food Safety and Standards Authority of India (FSSAI) norms, and has adequate toilet facilities. It is the responsibility of the hospital administration to maintain a safe environment for all of its patients, including cleanliness and offering infection control measures. Every patient has the right to get medical treatment that complies with the National Accreditation Board for Hospitals (NABH) or equivalent standards, norms, and standard operating procedures. They have a right to attention, treatment, and care that is professional, done with due care, and wholly under medical ethics. In the event of alleged medical malpractice or injury brought on by willful service delivery deficiencies, patients, and caregivers have the right to file a compensation claim. In line with the current care standards and accepted treatment protocols, the hospital administration, and treating physicians are obligated to deliver quality care. They also have a responsibility to prevent any form of medical malpractice or deficiency in the system for delivering services.

10. **Right to Choose Alternative Treatment Option if Available:** If there are alternative options for the treatment or management, patients and caretakers have the right to select one after carefully weighing all the possible alternatives. The patient and his or her caregivers would be responsible for any consequences if the patient chose to refuse care after carefully weighing all of his or her options. The observance of the different rights stated in this charter should not be impacted by a patient's independent decision to leave a hospital against medical advice, no matter how it may affect the patient's subsequent treatment or condition. The administration of the hospital has a responsibility to tell patients

about possible alternatives and respect their informed decisions with sufficient documentation and appropriate acknowledgment from patients or caregivers regarding the communication and approach.

11. **Right to Choose Source for Obtaining Medicines or Test:** Patients and caregivers are free to purchase any medication that has been prescribed by a physician from any registered pharmacy of their interest. When a specific diagnostic test is written by a physician, the patient and caretakers have the right to get it done from any authorized laboratory with trained personnel that is accredited by the National Accreditation Board for Laboratories (NABL). Every treating physician and hospital administration has a responsibility to let the patient and those who are caring for him know that they are free to get the required tests and medications from any pharmacy or diagnostic facility of their choosing. The treatment being offered by the concerned physician or clinical facility must not be adversely affected in any way by the patient's or caregiver's decision to use the pharmacy or diagnostic center of their choice.

12. **Right to Proper Referral and Transfer, this is Free from Perverse Commercial Influences:** Patients have a right to ongoing medical attention and the right to be properly registered at both the initial treatment center where treatment was sought and any additional facilities where care may be received. When transferring from one hospital or clinic to another, the patient or family members must be given a thorough explanation of the reasons behind the transfer, be informed of any available alternatives, and be given assurances that the transfer will be accepted by the receiving treatment center. Any requirements for ongoing medical care after hospital discharge must be disclosed to the patient and any carers by the hospital. The hospital management is responsible for making sure that patients are properly referred and transferred in the event of such a change in the treatment. Regarding all patient referrals, including those to other hospitals, specialists, laboratories, and imaging services, the decision regarding the facility to which the patient is referred must be based solely on the patient's best interests. There must be no commercial influence on the referral process such as incentives, commissions, and any other unethical tactics.

13. **Right to Protection for Patients Involved in Clinical Trials:** Everyone who is contacted to take part in a clinical study has the right to appropriate protection in this situation. All studies/

research must be carried out under adequate methodologies and good clinical practice recommendations. This includes adhering to the following client rights requirements:

a. Patient's participation in clinical studies must always be based on their express, freely given consent, after they have been fully informed of the risks and benefits of participating. The patient must receive a signed informed consent form, which serves as a document of the trial's basic information and serves as a legal record to support their willingness to participate in the study.

b. Participant's choice to consent to or deny participation in a clinical study must be honored, and their decision should not have an impact on standard medical treatments.

c. The name of the medication or intervention being studied, as well as the dates, dosage, and period of administration, should also be provided to the patient in writing.

d. A trial participant's privacy must always be protected, and all data obtained about the participant must be kept in strict confidence.

e. Participants in a clinical study who experience any adverse impact have the right to get the free medical care of adverse incidence, regardless of the injury's relationship to the clinical trial, for as long as necessary or until it is determined that the harm is unrelated to the research study. In addition, they must receive financial or other support to make up for any impairment or disability. Their immediate family members are entitled to compensation in the event of death.

f. During the duration of a clinical trial, participants may get ancillary care for conditions unrelated to the study or trial. Depending on the circumstances, this could involve medical care or facility referrals.

g. Institutional measures must be put in place to permit insurance coverage for illnesses related to or unrelated to the study (ancillary care) and the payment of compensation whenever the relevant ethics committee seems necessary.

h. Participants in the experiment should be guaranteed access to the best treatment options, which the study may have demonstrated.

It is the responsibility of any medical practitioner or medical center that is associated with a clinical trial to make certain that all of these standards are adhered to if any individuals or patients participate in a study.

14. **Right to Protection of Participants Involved in Biomedical and Health Research:** Everyone who participates in the biomedical study is called a "research participant," and everyone who is a research participant has the right to be protected. Any trial/study carried out among such participants must adhere to the National Ethical Guidelines for Biomedical and Health Research Involving Human Participants, 2017 established by the Indian Council of Medical Research, and be conducted with the Ethics Committee's prior approval. The research subject's signed informed consent should be obtained. Research involving a vulnerable group should be conducted with additional safety precautions. Individual's and community's rights to secrecy, privacy, and dignity should be upheld.

    If research participants are harmed in any way—physical, mental, social, legal, or economic—due to their participation, they are entitled to receive financial or other support in fairly and equal manner for any temporary or long-term illness or disability. When applicable, individuals, groups, and societies should have access to the benefits that result from the study.

15. **Right to take Discharge of Patient, or Receive Body of Deceased from Hospital:** All patients have the right to be discharged and cannot be held against their will in a hospital for procedural reasons such as a disagreement over medical bill payment. Similar to this, primary caregivers have the right to the deceased body of a hospital-treated patient, and the deceased body cannot be withheld for procedural reasons such as failing to pay or a disagreement over payment of medical bills in opposition to the preferences of the caregivers. The hospital administration has a responsibility to uphold these rights and not, under any circumstances, engage in the wrongful imprisonment of any patient or patient's dead body who has received medical attention there.

16. **Right to Patient Education:** Every patient has the right to learn important information about their status and better and healthier ways to live, as well as their rights and duties, health insurance plans issued by the government that apply to them, and their rights and responsibilities in the case of nonprofit hospitals, and the way for their problems fixed in the language they understand or ask for the information. The administration of the facility and concerning physician has a responsibility to give each patient this instruction under the normal protocol, using language that the patients can understand.

17. **Right to be Heard and Seek Redressal:** Every patient has the right to provide comments about the medical care they are currently receiving from a physician or facility, as well as to voice any concerns they may have with that care. A key part of this is the right to clear and straightforward instructions and guidance on how to provide input in the form of suggestions, complaints, or other types of feedback. This can be executed by filing a complaint with a duly authorized healthcare facility for this purpose, as well as with a formal mechanism established by the government, such as the Patients' Rights Tribunal Forum, depending on the situation. Every complaint must be required to register by issuing a registration number, and there must be a trustable track-trace system in place so that it can be determined how far along the complaint investigation process it is. A fair and timely resolution of the patient's and the caregivers' complaints is assured. They also have the right to obtain the complaint's resolution in writing within 15 days of the day it was received. Under the Patient's Rights Charter, every clinical facility and hospital is required to establish an internal redress system and to enforce compliance and cooperate fully with official redress systems. This entails providing all pertinent information and acting entirely under the redress body's directives.

Responsibilities of Patients and Caretakers

Patients and caregivers should uphold their obligations in addition to advocating for their rights so that medical facilities and practitioners can do their jobs effectively.

- ❖ To facilitate diagnosis and treatment, patients should provide their physicians with all necessary health-related information in response to the physician's questions, without concealing pertinent information.
- ❖ Patients need to remember that it is their right to be involved in the decision-making process regarding their treatment, but they also need to cooperate with their doctors during the assessment, laboratory studies, and treatment, and they need to follow their advice.
- ❖ Patients are expected to adhere to all scheduling instructions, cooperate with medical personnel and other patients, refrain from disturbing other patients, and keep the hospital clean.

- Patients should respect the medical staff's dignity both as professionals and as human beings. Whatever the complaint, patients and caregivers must refrain from using violence of any kind and from damaging or destroying hospital or service provider property.
- Patients must accept responsibility for their actions, both if they choose not to receive treatment and based on those decisions.

CHAPTER HIGHLIGHTS

- The International Council of Nurses (ICN) first ratified a global code of ethics for nurses in 1953.
- The *ICN Code of Ethics for Nurses* has four principal elements that provide a framework for ethical conduct.
- The 1948 Universal Declaration of Human Rights places a strong emphasis on the inherent dignity and equality of every person.
- Various legal provisions of patient's rights are dispersed throughout various legal documents in India.
- There are 17 patient rights described by the Ministry of Health and family welfare Government of India.

MULTIPLE CHOICE QUESTIONS

1. In which year, did the International Council of Nurses (ICN) first approve a global code of ethics for nurses?
   a. 1953
   b. 1952
   c. 1951
   d. 1950
2. Which of the following is not an element of the code of ethics by the International Council of Nurses (ICN)?
   a. Nurses and the global health
   b. Nurses and the practice
   c. Nurses and the profession
   d. Nurses and the culture
3. "The nurse respects the uniqueness of the individual in the provision of care." This statement is an element of the code of ethics by which regulatory body?
   a. International Council of Nurses (ICN)
   b. Trained nurses' association of India (TNAI)
   c. National Institute of Health (NIH)
   d. Indian Nursing Council
4. In which year, the Ministry of Health and Family Welfare, Government of India published the first "Charter of Patient Rights"?
   a. 1946
   b. 2016
   c. 2017
   d. 2018

5. How many fundamental rights are listed in the Ministry of Health and Family Welfare (MoHFW; 2018), 'Charter of Patients Rights'?
   a. 15
   b. 16
   c. 17
   d. 18

ANSWERS

1. a   2. d   3. d   4. d   5. c

■ BIBLIOGRAPHY

1. Blackwood S, Chiarella M. Barriers to uptake and use of codes of ethics by nurses. Collegian. 2020;27(4):443-9.
2. Channabasavanna SM, Murthy P. The National human rights Commission report 1999: a defining moment. In: Agarwal SP (Ed). Mental health: An Indian perspective 1946–2003. Gurugram: Elsevier; 2004:108-12.
3. Ghooi RB, Deshpande SR. Patients' rights in India: an ethical perspective. Indian J Med Ethics. 2012;9(4):277-81.
4. Kumar TD. Unfolding the theme: Human Rights and Nurses' Role. Nursing Journal of India. 2005;96(12):281.
5. Sharma S. Human rights of mental patients in India: a global perspective. Curr Opin Psychiatry. 2003;16(5):547-51.
6. Singh JA, Govender M, Mills EJ. Do human rights matter to health? Lancet. 2007;370(9586):521-7.
7. Stievano A, Tschudin V. The ICN code of ethics for nurses: a time for revision. Int Nurs Rev. 2019;66(2):154-6.
8. Suresh S. Nursing research and statistics, 3rd edition. Gurugram: Elsevier Health Sciences; 2018.
9. Thompson HO, Thompson JE. Code of ethics for nurse-midwives. J Nurse Midwifery. 1986;31(2):99-102.
10. Zahedi F, Sanjari M, Aala M, Peymani M, Aramesh K, Parsapour A, et al. The code of ethics for nurses. Iran J Public Health. 2013;42(Supple1):1-8.

Index

Page numbers followed by *f* refer to figure and *t* refer to table.

A

Abortion 130, 131
  debate 131
Accountability 6, 114
Achievement 69
Active euthanasia 147
Adaptability 33
Advocacy 20, 100
  benefits of 102
  ill effects of 102
  types of 100
Affective empathy 84
Allow natural death 143, 144
Alternative decisions, identification of 161
Alternative search 67
Altruism 16, 70, 82, 85
  drawbacks of 86
  types of 85
Altruistic behaviors, characteristics of 85
American Nurses Association 113, 150
Assisted dying 147
Assisted reproductive technologies 139, 140, 140*f*
  types of 140
Assisted suicide 148
Autonomy 6, 16, 19, 30, 70, 109

B

Behavioral empathy 84
Beneficence 30, 111
Benevolence 70
Bioethics 105, 107, 108
Body language 29

C

Caregiver 11, 47
Caretakers, responsibilities of 187
Caring 9, 78
  behaviour, importance of 81
  characteristics of 79
  components of 79
  five C's of 80*f*
Client advocate 12
Clinical decision making 165
Clinical Establishment Act 179
Code of ethics 5, 16, 113, 170, 171*f*, 175
  adherence to 22
Code, purpose of 37, 171
Cognitive empathy 83
Collaboration 21
Collect additional information 159
Collegiality 21
Communication 24, 39
  challenges 43
  skills 9
Communicator 11
Community service 23
Compassionate care 80
Competence 23, 80
Computerized provider order entry 127
Confidence 81
Confidentiality 93-95, 122
  essential components of 94*f*
Conflicts concerning new technologies 127
Conformity 69
Conscientiousness 86
  characteristics of 87
Consequences, awareness of 85
Consumer Protection Act 179
Context-related issues 32
Continuous professional growth 8
Contraceptive 138
Courageousness 80
COVID-19 101, 110
Credibility 98
Cultivate existing conscientious habit 88

D

Deception 121
Decision making, autonomy in 70
Dedication, outcomes of 90
Devotion 89
Dominant values 65
Donor
  eggs 141
  sperm 141

Double effect, principle of 145
Drugs and Cosmetics Act 179

E

Economic security 8, 19
Education 25
Electronic health record 127, 128
Electronic medical record 127
Embryo 140
    development time 141
    selection 142
    storage, time limit for 142
Emergency medical care 181
Emotional component 80
Empathetic nursing practices 84
Empathy 10, 82
    components of 83, 83f
Ethical decision-making 162, 157
    model 161f, 162t
        application of 161
        process 158, 159f, 160
    process 158
        significance of 157
Ethical dilemma 118, 122, 126, 127, 131, 135, 138, 141, 158
Ethical issues 118, 136, 137
Ethical principles 40, 42t, 109, 110, 133, 160
    application of 109
    summary of 110t
    violation of 152
Ethical theories 108t
Ethics 21, 105, 107
    code of 5, 16, 113, 170, 171f, 175
    committee 163
        responsibilities of 165
        role of 165
    fundamental principles of 41f
Euthanasia 147
    types of 147, 148f
Extrinsic values 65

F

Factors affecting
    altruism 86
    professional socialization 73
Factors influencing dedication 89
Falsifying records 27
Feelings, encourage verbal expression of 101
Fetal
    alcohol
        spectrum disorders 133
        syndrome 133
    conditions, intrauterine treatment of 134
    conflict 134
    injury 138
    therapy 134, 135
Fidelity 98, 113
    effect of 99
Forced choice rank 66
Forensic nurse 13
Frozen sperm, use of 142
Fundamental ethical principles 109t

G

Genetic
    altruism 85
    screening 142
Group-selected altruism 85

H

Hastening death 145
Health care 77
Hedonism 69
Honesty 96
Human dignity 70, 92, 101
    aspects of 91
    maintenance of 93
    respect for 30, 91
Human immunodeficiency virus 139, 163, 183
Human sense of 10

I

Implement decision 160
Implementation 161
In utero harm 138
In vitro fertilization 135, 140
Inclusive language, use of 29
Indian Medical Council 16, 18, 52, 179, 175
Indian Nursing Council
    functions of 52
    organizational structure of 52f
Indian Professional Nursing Organizations 56
Indian Society of Psychiatric Nurses 56, 58
Infertility treatment 139, 141
Informed consent 31, 124, 126
Innovation 20
Integration 71, 75, 76
Integrity 96
Intellectual activities 15
Interest, conflict of 119, 120
International Confederation of Midwives 54, 55

Index

International Council of Nurses 16, 54, 170
   code 171
   elements of 171*f*
   functions of 55
   objectives of 55
International Federation of Perioperative Nurses 54, 56
International Professional Organizations 54
International Society of Mental Health Nursing and Allied Health Professionals 58
Intracytoplasmic sperm injection 140
Intrauterine
   devices 137
   insemination 140
Intrinsic values 65
Issues concerning consent 162

J

Job-related factors 90
Joint commission 152

K

Kantianism 108
Knowledge
   body of 15
   intellectual and body of 7

L

Leadership 10
Legal obligations 115
Life-sustaining treatment 144
   medical order for 144, 145

M

Maintaining altruistic behaviour, benefits of 86
Maternal conflict 134
Medical Termination of Pregnancy Act 130
Mission 54, 56
Moral empathy 84
Moral obligations 115
Morality 107, 108
Motivation 76
Multiple gestations 140

N

National Accreditation Board for Hospitals 183
National Human Rights Commission 180
Non-maleficence 30, 111
Non-therapeutic touch 47

Nurse 113, 176, 177, 178
   administrator 13
   devotion of 89
   educator 13
   entrepreneur 13
   informatics 13
   midwife 13
   practitioner 12
   qualities of 9, 9*f*
   researcher 13
   responsibility of 11, 11*f*, 98, 148
   role of 11, 11*f*, 125, 126
Nurses League of Christian Medical Association of India 56
Nursing 1, 14, 70, 90
   education, advocacy for 100, 101
   practice 27, 38, 81, 110*t*
   profession
      characteristics of 13, 14*f*
      criteria of 15
   professional in 1
   requires personal contact 14
Obligations 115
   types of 115*f*
Occupation 4, 5, 5*t*
Open communication 29
Oral contraceptives 137
Palliative sedation 146
Passive euthanasia 148
Paternalism 120
Patient's rights 102
Patient's rights 150, 170, 179
   charter of 180*f*
Patient's
   advocacy for 100, 101
   responsibilities of 187
Personal development 8
Personal values 69, 75*f*, 76
   integration of 71, 75
Personnel protective equipment, adequate supply of 101
Physical component 79
Physician assisted suicide 147
Positive values 65
Posture 44
Power 69
Pregnancy, termination of 130
Privacy 92-95, 122
   essential components of 94*f*
Profession 3-5, 5*t*, 8
   Bixler's criteria for 7*f*
   characteristics of 5, 5*f*
   criteria of 6
   Flexner's criteria of 6*f*

Professional 1
   advancement 40
   boundary 47
      violation 47
   competency 71
   conduct 36, 40
      code of 37, 37t, 41f, 177
   etiquettes 44
   grooming 45
   identity 24, 25
   issues 102
   organization 24, 51, 53
      importance of 54, 72
   relationship 47
      continuum of 47f
   responsibility 37
   socialization 71
   standards 5
   values 61, 63, 69, 70, 75f, 77, 77f
      importance of 77
      integration of 71, 75
Professionalism 3, 16, 17, 22, 157
   attributes of 19, 20f
   challenges of 24, 25
   characteristics of 17, 18f
   concepts of 21, 22f
   indicators of 21
   Miller's wheel of 21
Psychiatric care 151
Psychological component 80
Reciprocal altruism 85
Regulatory bodies 51
   purposes of 51f
Research development 23
Research ethics committees 163
   basic responsibilities of 164
   members 164
   role of 166
Restraints, types of 153
Role confusion 25

S

Scarce health resources, allocation of 126
Security 69
Self-confidence 91
Self-determination 18
Self-integrity
   importance of 27
   preservation of 25

Self-regulation 18, 23
Sexually transmitted disease 110
Sharing personal information 47
State Nursing Council 53
   functions of 53
Stimulation 69
Student Nurses' Association of
      India 56-58
   activities of 58
   key activities of 58f
Substance abuse
   during pregnancy 132
   major complications of 133t
Support systems 44
Sympathy 71, 82, 141

T

Team members 47
Terminal sedation 146
Theory development and utilization 23
Trained Nurses' Association of
      India 16, 56
Truth-telling 30, 96, 122

U

Unprofessional language, use of 45t

V

Values 21
   characteristics of 64
   clarification 65, 65f
      strategies for 66
   congruence 76
   continuum 67
   formation 68
   neutrality 67
   types of 65
   voting 67
Variant values 65
Veracity 112
Virtue ethics 108
Vision 55, 56

W

Whistleblowing 128, 129
Withdrawing medical intervention 142
Withholding information 26
Work atmosphere 86
Work environment, advocacy for 100, 101

EU GSPR Authorised Reprsentative
Logos Europe, 9 rue Nicolas Poussin
1700, La Rochelle, France
Phone: +33 (0) 6 67 93 73 78
E-mail: contact@logoseurope.eu

www.ingramcontent.com/pod-product-compliance
Ingram Content Group UK Ltd.
Pitfield, Milton Keynes, MK11 3LW, UK
UKHW021831140426
5217IPUK00021B/1391